LOW FODMAP DIET FOR BEGINNERS

Discover Proven Soothing Recipes and Elimination Diet for Fast IBS Relief, Digestive Disorders, Vegan Gut and Bloat Problems

Mollie Capalino, Sue Tunitsky, and Kate Shepherd

James Shepherd

Danielle Scarlet

Table of Contents

PART 1

Chapter 1: Introduction to the Low FODMAP diet

Do you suffer from abdominal cramping and discomfort? If you spend your days feeling constipated, bloated, and feel the uncontrollable urge to use the bathroom? If so, you may suffer from IBS.

With so many diets on the market, it can be hard to decide which one is best for you! In the following chapters, you will be learning everything you need to know about the FODMAP diet and how it can benefit your life.

Unfortunately, there are several theories behind why individuals suffer from IBS. For many, there is 70% of women who suffer from IBS due to their hormones triggering the symptoms. As for others, the reasons could be anything from a sensitive colon, an immune response to stressors, sensitive brain activity in detecting gut contractions, or even a neurotransmitter serotonin being produced in the gut. While the doctors are unable to pinpoint an exact reason for IBS, the good news is that they are certain that IBS will not cause other gastrointestinal diseases and it is not cancer!

The right question to ask in this moment, is what can I do about it? We are here to tell you that the low FODMAP diet is the way to go. In the chapters to follow, you will learn everything from what the diet is, who the diet is for, what FODMAP even stands for, and why this diet will work for you. We cover the benefits of the diet and include an easy start guide so you can get rid of that discomfort and bloat as soon as possible!

To start, it is important to understand what the FODMAP diet is, and why it is something you need to start. However, before we start, here are some tips for the beginners who are just starting or considering the low FODMAP diet.

Getting Started

Before we begin, it is important to get a diagnosis from your family doctor. Many people self-diagnose themselves with IBS and place themselves on the low FODMAP diet. This is something we do not recommend. If you have symptoms such as pain and bloating, you should see a professional to rule out any possible life-threatening diseases.

What is IBS?

As mentioned, be sure to see a professional to attain an official prognosis of IBS. If you suspect you do have Irritable Bowel Syndrome, realize that you are not alone. In fact, around 15% of the population in the United States suffer from IBS symptoms. While the symptoms do vary from person to person, the typical symptoms are as follow:

- Bloating
- Constipation
- Diarrhea
- Lower Abdominal Pain
- Lower Abdominal Discomfort

If you suffer from any of these, it is important to consult with your doctor the specific symptoms you have. This will be vital as there are three different types of irritable bowel syndrome. These include:

- IBS with Constipation
  - Typically, IBS with constipation has symptoms including bloating, abnormally delayed bowel movements, stomach pains, and loose or lumpy stool.
- IBS with Diarrhea
  - Typically comes with symptoms including stomach pain, urgent need to use the bathroom, loose and watery stool
- IBS with alternating Diarrhea and Constipation

Due to the fact that there are several types of IBS, this makes it hard to determine a single drug treatment to help with the symptoms. As we mentioned earlier, you need to consult with a professional. Once you have done this and ruled out any other illnesses, it is time to take a look at your diet.

Who is the diet for?

Typically, the low FODMAP diet is meant for individuals suffering from IBS. The diet itself was created as one of the first food-based treatments to help relieve IBS symptoms. The good news is that up to 75% of patients who had IBS experienced symptom relief when they followed the low FODMAP diet. However, the diet is also helpful if you have any of the following:

- Digestive Disorder
  - Gastroesophageal Reflux Disease (GERD)
  - Crohn's Disease
  - Celiac Disease

- Vegan Gut
- Bloating

Once you have determined that the low FODMAP diet could help your symptoms, it is now time to learn what FODMAP even stands for! This is going to be vital information to carry with you through your diet so you understand what you are eating and why your body is reacting the way it does!

We understand that there are many different types of diets out there. Some of you may be wondering, can I follow my current diet and still follow the low FODMAP diet? The answer varies depending on which you follow, and we will try to answer in a simple manner:

- Vegetarian/ Vegan
  - o Yes, this diet is more than possible to follow if you are vegan or vegetarian. With a few tweaks, you can find friendly options and still stick to your regular diet!
- Low-Salt
  - o If you follow a low-salt diet, this diet is doable for you. However, it will be vital that you learn how to read and follow food labels. Luckily for you, this is information also included in this book!
- Gluten-Free
  - o As you will be learning, the FODMAP diet does exclude wheat, which contains gluten. If you are gluten-free, this diet is easy to follow as you most likely will not be able to have it anyway!

- Kosher
  - If you have to eat kosher, you can still follow this diet. It will be up to you to find certain kosher foods, but after the elimination diet, you will be able to find the foods and still stick to your original diet.

History of the low FODMAP diet

Originally, the low FODMAP diet was developed by a team of scientists at the Monash University located in Australia. The original research was meant to investigate if the diet would be able to control IBS symptoms with food alone. The university established a food analysis program to study FODMAPs in both Australian as well as international foods.

In 2005, the first FODMAP ideas would be published as part of a research paper. In the paper, the hypothesis was that by reducing dietary intake of certain foods that were deemed indigestible, this could help reduce symptoms stimulated in an individual's gut's nervous system.

Over many years, research has shown that certain short-chain carbohydrates such as lactose, sorbitol, and fructose was the cause behind gastrointestinal discomfort. Once the basis of digestion was studied, the low FODMAP diet was created to help with these symptoms.

What does FODMAP stand for?

FODMAPs are typically found in foods that we consume every day. They are in onions, rye, barley, wheat, garlic, milk, fruits, vegetables, and more! As you can tell from this very small list (don't worry, we will cover more in the chapters to follow), they are in some of our more common foods! This is why it is so easy to feel bloated for some people, without understanding what is causing it! However, before we dive into how this diet works, you will need to understand the acronym FODMAP.

F-Fermentable

O- Oligosaccharies (short chain carbohydrates)

D- Disaccharides (lactose)

M- Monosaccharides (fructose)

A- and

P- Polyols (Sorbitol, xylitol, maltitol, and mannitol)

The reason you may be suffering from IBS or other digestive issues is due to the fact that most FODMAPs have a hard time absorbing into your small intestine. As a result, these FODMAPs are fermented by the bacteria in your small and large intestine in which results in bloating and irregular bowel movements.

While the FODMAPs cause the digestive discomfort, it is important to understand that it is not the cause of the intestinal inflammation itself. In fact, the FODMAPs produce alterations of intestinal flora that help you maintain a healthy colon. This does not change that the symptoms are still uncomfortable.

What may be causing your IBS symptoms could be a fructose malabsorption or a lactose intolerance. As you will be learning in later chapters, as you begin the low FODMAP diet, there will be an elimination phase where you learn what exactly is causing your symptoms and discomfort.

The source of the FODMAP will vary depending on different dietary groups. In more common circumstances they are compromised as the following:

- Oligosaccharies: Fructans and Galacto-oligosaccharies
- Disaccharies- Lactose
- Monosaccharies- Fructose
- Polyols- Xylitol, Mannitol, Sorbitol

Sources of Fructans

In later chapters, we will be going more in-depth on the foods you can and cannot eat. To cover the basics, you should understand where these specific irritants come from. To start, we will go over the source of fructans. These can be found in very popular ingredients including; rye, garlic, onion, wheat, beetroot, Brussel sprouts, and certain prebiotics.

Sources of Galactans

As for galactans, these are primarily found in beans and pulses. It can also be found in certain tofu and tempeh, but this does not mean that vegans and vegetarians cannot follow the low FODMAP diet. It simply means that you will need to find other sources of proteins if you want to follow a plant-based diet. We will be going over this more in the chapters to follow.

Sources of Polyols

Polyols are typically found in stone fruits. These include avocados, apples, blackberries, watermelon, and more. They are also found naturally in certain vegetables and bulk sweeteners.

While this diet may seem to be lacking many of your favorite foods, don't you worry! Due to the wide variety of IBS symptoms, it is unclear which foods trigger certain individuals. This is why the elimination trial will be important before you start the diet. Please remember that everyone is different. While some people see immediate results when they begin the diet, for others, it will take some time.

Effectiveness and Risks of the low FODMAP diet

It is important to understand that the low FODMAP diet is meant for short-term symptom relief. However, long-term diet can have a negative effect on your body. Unfortunately, it can be detrimental to your guy metabolome and microbiota. It is to be taken very seriously that this diet is meant for short periods of time and only under the advice of a professional.

Please understand that if you choose to follow the low FODMAP diet without any medical advice, it is possible the diet could lead to some serious health risks. Some of these risks are as followed:

- Nutritional Deficiencies
- Increased Risk of Cancer
- Death

When you start the low FODMAP diet, it is possible the diet itself could mask any serious disease that present themselves of digestive symptoms. These could include celiac disease, colon cancer, or inflammatory bowel disease. This is why it is so crucial to seek professional help before starting the diet on your own.

Now that you have learned the basics of the low FODMAP diet, it is time to learn all about the benefits that come with the diet change. Obviously, the main change will be to help lower any digestive troubles you may behaving. By removing the potential triggers in which are causing your digestive issues, this will help pinpoint which food intolerances you have.

While this diet may seem to take a lot of time and effort, think of the time you are wasting by being in discomfort all of the time and using the bathroom! With a few minor adjustments and tests, you will be able to find the source of your problem and hopefully never feel this way again! Now, onto learn all of the other incredible benefits the low FODMAP diet can bring to you!

Chapter 2: Benefits of the Low FODMAP diet

According to research, the low FODMAP diet is effective for around 75% of patients who suffer from IBS. In most cases, the patients are able reduce any major symptoms they are experiencing and in hand, improve their quality of life.

In the same research, scientist found evidence that the diet can also be beneficial for people who suffer from other functional gastrointestinal disorders such as Chron's disease, ulcerative colitis, and inflammatory bowel disease. All you need to do to benefit from this diet is to figure out what is causing the digestive disturbances and symptoms. Below, you will find some of the other benefits the low FODMAP diet has to offer:

A. IBS Symptom Reduction

By following the low FODMAP diet, individuals can reduce most symptoms involved with IBS including stomach pain, bloating, and gas. It is important to follow the diet and remove any irritants as they ferment inside of your intestines. By selecting foods that don't trigger your symptoms, you can avoid them altogether!

B. Chron's Disease Reduced Discomfort
By following the low FODMAP diet, individuals were able to change the quality and number of prebiotics. By controlling the foods you consume and avoiding the ones that trigger your system, you could reduce the discomfort you feel from the trigger foods.

C. Increased Energy

Some individuals feel tired no matter how much they eat through the day. It is believed that a low FODMAP diet can help reduce fatigue. This could be due to the fact that the body is no longer wasting energy on digesting foods that don't agree with your system. This is especially true for sweeteners that you could be using on a daily basis. As you will be learning later, some of the best sweeteners can be found in fruit!

D. Reduced Constipation and Diarrhea

When you follow the low FODMAP diet, you will begin to eliminate foods that are causing your symptoms in the first place. When you do this, your body will find a balance, and you may find that your bloating will decrease, the gas will decrease, and your stools will return to normal. It is a win-win situation! All you will need to do is figure out your triggers (which we cover in the third chapter) and follow the diet!

On top of these incredible benefits, there is also beliefs that the low FODMAP diet can benefit psychological health. Often times, the disturbances of IBS can cause stress to certain individuals, eventually leading to anxiety and depression. When you remove the trigger causing the symptoms by diet, you will be able to improve the quality of your life.

As you will be learning in the chapters to follow, the low FODMAP diet includes an elimination diet in order to get started. As you introduce foods, you may find that you have a lactose or gluten intolerance. While this may seem like a huge change, there are some incredible benefits to changing your diet.

Benefits of a Grain Free Diet

As you will be learning later in the book, there are many types of grains that has been found to cause inflammation. Unfortunately, this is a very common culprit for the digestive disorders you may be experiencing. This is especially true if you are very sensitive to gluten. The good news is that if you are looking to lose weight on top of feeling better, cutting out these grains will be the best thing to ever happen to you. Reined grains are high in carbohydrates and calories; they offer little to no nutrition and contribute to discomfort in your stomach. Before you make the switch to going grain free, consider some of the amazing benefits as follow:

A. Digestion Benefits

Gluten is a type of protein that can be found in wheat products. If you do the elimination diet and find that you are gluten sensitive, cutting it out makes the most sense. When you cut it out of your diet, this can help relieve issues such as nausea, bloating, diarrhea and constipation.

B. Reduced Inflammation

When you experience acute inflammation, this normally means that your immune system is fighting off foreign invaders. Unfortunately, if you sustain these levels for a long period of time, this is what causes chronic disease. By cutting gluten out, you can reduce the amount of inflammation in your body.

C. Balanced Microbiome

By following a grain-free diet, you will be able to balance the microbiome in your gut. When you do this, it helps support the beneficial bacteria in your body, helping improve your digestion, boost your immunity, and helps keep blood sugar under control.

D. Weight Loss

As mentioned earlier, most grains offer little to no nutrition. When you cut these extra calories out of your diet, it will help you lose weight. Instead of grains, try eating nutrient-dense foods like vegetables or legumes. Of course, you will figure out exactly what you can eat on the low FODMAP diet after going through the elimination portion.

Another common irritant when individuals suffer from IBS and other digestive orders can be lactose! You may be thinking to yourself; I could never give up my yogurt or ice cream. The good news is that in the current market, some incredible alternative choices can fit in the low FODMAP diet. In case you need some further benefits to help convince you, here are just a few:

E. Healthier Digestion

You may not know, but around 70% of the population has a degrees of intolerance to lactose. When we first begin to wean off of our mother's milk, we begin to use lactase. Lactase is an enzyme that helps digest lactose found in milk. As we age, we begin to lose the ability to digest lactose and is one of the biggest known triggers for IBS. By taking dairy out of your diet, you save yourself the troubles all together!

F. Decreased Bloating

Bloating occurs when we have issues with digestion. Some dairy products can cause excessive gas in the intestines, which is what causes the bloating in the first place. Some bodies are unable to break down the carbohydrates and sugar fully which in turn, creates an imbalance of gut bacteria.

G. Clearer Skin

If you suffer from acne, dairy could be the culprit! According to studies posted in Clinics in Dermatology, it was found that dairy products such as milk contain growth hormones that stimulate acne. By following the low FODMAP diet and cutting dairy from your diet, you could naturally treat acne!

H. Reduce Risk of Cancer

A 2001 study at Harvard School of Public Health found that there was a connection between high calcium intake and increased risk of prostate cancer. It is thought that the hormones in the milk contain contaminants such as pesticides that have been linked to cancer cell growth. These contaminants are mostly found in dairy products, giving you another reason to cut them from your diet altogether!

I. Decreased Oxidative Stress

It is believed that a high milk intake is typically associated with higher mortality rates in both men and women. This may be due to the D-galatose found in milk which helps influence oxidative stress and inflammation in the body. Unfortunately, this undesirable effect caused by milk can cause chronic expose and damage health. On top of inflammation, it can also shorten life spans, cause neurodegeneration and also decrease one's immune system.

As you can tell, there are so many incredible benefits of switching over to the low FODMAP diet. Whether you are looking to get rid of bloating, lose some weight, or stop constipation and/or diarrhea, the low FODMAP diet has got you covered. It is all a matter of figuring out what your trigger is in the first place.

Obviously, we could go on and on about the incredible benefits of the diet, but then we would never get to the diet itself! Now that you are aware of just some of the benefits, it is time to get you started! In the chapter to follow, you will be learning how to get started on the low FODMAP diet. You will the steps to get started on the diet itself and how to diet whether you are vegan, vegetarian, diabetics, or doing this for a child who suffers from IBS. When you are ready, we can dive in!

Chapter 3: Starting the Low FODMAP diet

Now that you are aware of the low FODMAP diet and some of its benefits, it is time to learn how you can get started on the diet yourself! While a diet and lifestyle change can seem daunting, it will be important to believe in yourself and remember why you started it in the first place. In the chapter to follow, we will be providing you with all of the information you need. From diagnosis of IBS, to starting the diet, and even how to practice if you are vegan, vegetarian, or diabetic. This diet can be universal; it is all about finding what works best for you. First, it is time to understand the diagnosis of IBS.

Getting Diagnosed with IBS and FODMAP Tests

If you are in the process of being diagnosed with a chronic medical condition, this could be a challenging time for you. It is important that you understand the symptoms the doctors are looking for, and which medical tests you will be taking in order to be officially diagnosed with irritable bowel syndrome. IBS can be diagnosed with a combination of Rome IV criteria so the doctors will be able to rule out any other gastrointestinal disorders.

Rome IV is a set of criteria that doctors have found that most IBS patients have in common. This criteria is 98% accurate when the doctors are identifying their patients with IBS. These criteria are as followed:

1. Recurrent abdominal pain at least one day per week in the last three months are have the following:

    A. Related to defecation

B. A change in stool frequency

C. Change in form of stool

2. Criteria from above is fulfilled with symptoms for at least six months before official diagnosis

Other symptoms often associated with IBS include bloating, abdominal pain, and a change in bowel habit. Your doctor will take in the evidence and match with the Rome IV criteria and will move onto discussing any red flag symptoms that may be occurring.

Before being diagnosed with IBS, it will be important that your doctor rules out any other medical conditions that could be presented with the same symptoms; this is where the red flag symptoms come into play. These flags include:

- Inflammatory Markers
- Rectal Masses
- Abdominal Masses
- Anemia
- Nocturnal Symptoms such as waking up from sleep to defecate
- Family History of coeliac disease, inflammatory bowel disease, and ovarian cancer
- Rectal Bleeding
- Unintentional Weight Loss

On top of these symptoms, your doctor will also ask for several other symptoms in order to diagnose you with IBS. Firstly, the discomfort and pain in your abdomen will need to be related to altered bowel frequency as well as a change in your stool form. You will also need to have at least two of the following symptoms:

1. Feeling incomplete emptying when using the bathroom
2. Passage of mucus when using the bathroom
3. Straining, Urgency, and Altered Stool passage
4. Abdominal Bloating
5. Lethargy
6. Backaches
7. Bladder Symptoms
8. Nausea

Medical Tests for IBS

Once your doctor figures out your symptoms, rules out any other serious medical conditions and believes it is appropriate to run tests for IBS can you expect one of the following tests:

- Antibody testing for coeliac disease
- C-reactive protein
- Erythrocyte sedimentation rate
- Full blood count

While these tests are typical, it may be different if you present any of the red flag symptoms from above. If you do have a red flag symptom, there will be additional tests to rule out any more serious issues. These tests are as follow:

- Hydrogen Breath Test (meant for lactose intolerance)
- Fecal Occult Blood

- Fecal Ova and Parasite Test
- Thyroid Function Test
- Rigid/ Flexible Sigmoidoscopy
- Ultrasound

In the case that your doctor feels your symptoms may not be linked to IBS, they will most likely refer you to a gastroenterologist. This is a physician who is an expert in managing diseases found in the liver and gastrointestinal tract. However, this is worst case scenario. For now, we will focus on following the diet if you are diagnosed with IBS.

Breaking down FODMAPS

In general, FODMAPs naturally occur in popular foods such as vegetables, fruits, grains, cereals, dairy products, and legumes. Unfortunately for those who suffer from IBS, these FODMAPs are absorbed poorly in our small intestines and can affect our bowels as a symptom. FODMAPs are short-chain carbohydrates found in these foods, but this does not mean that the diet itself is sugar-free. When we consume FODMAPs, they are fermented by gut bacteria in the large intestine in which triggers the unpleasant GI symptoms that you may be experiencing. Before we move onto the elimination stage, it is important to understand just what this acronym means.

Fermentable

Fermenting is the process where our gut bacteria attempt so break down FODMAPs. As you are already aware, these FODMAPs are indigestible carbohydrates and in turn, produce gas.

Oligo-Saccharies

This group of the FODMAP are broken down into two subgroups including fructans and galactans. Fructans also known as fructo-oligosaccharies or FOS are most commonly found in foods such as dried fruit, barley rye, wheat, garlic, onion. Galactans or galacto-oligosaccharies or GOS are found in pulses, legumes, cashews, pistachios, and silken tofu. If you feel yourself panicking over remembering these foods, don't worry. In the chapter to follow, we will cover exactly what you can and cannot eat while on the low FODMAP diet.

Di-Saccharies

As mentioned in the chapter from before, lactose could be a potential trigger in your diet. These can be found in any product that comes from goat, sheep, or cow's milk. Lactose itself contains two sugars united that require an enzyme known as lactase before our bodies are even able to absorb it. When your gut lacks these enzymes, this is when you can trigger symptoms of IBS.

Mono-Saccharides

This is a fructose that is found when a person has an excess amount of glucose in their diet. Our bodies need an equal amount of glucose in our system to stop any malabsorption. This means that while some of us can consume a certain amount of glucose, it is important to avoid foods that contain an excess amount. Some examples of these excessive foods include asparagus, honey, apples, and pears.

And Polyols

Polyols are also known as sugar alcohols. These can be found in a wide range of vegetables and fruits including sweet potatoes, mushrooms, pears, and apples. These sugar alcohols are also found artificial sweeteners in chewing gum, diabetic candy, and even protein powder. These polyols can only be partially absorbed into our small intestines. The rest continue into the large intestine, begin to ferment, and cause discomfort and bloating for some people.

As you begin to consider the low FODMAP diet, it is important to understand that one size does not fit all. This diet will change depending on your intolerance to certain foods. On the FODMAP diet, you will be following three different phases including: The Elimination Phase, The Reintroduction Phase, and the Maintenance Phase. We will go further into detail of each phase, so you have a full understanding before beginning.

The Elimination Phase

The Elimination phase is also known as the restriction phase. While this may seem intimidating, realize that this phase is only meant to last two to six weeks. This phase should only last long enough for you to gain control over your symptoms. Once this happens, you will move onto the reintroduction phase with the help of a professional. It is important that this stage is short as it can have long-term effects on your gut health.

To begin, you will want to create a personal list of foods you feel makes your IBS worse. If you are unsure which foods could be causing your symptoms, you will want to check out the next chapter to see an extended list of foods you should be avoiding. Some popular starters include chocolate, coffee, nuts, and certain fibers.

Once you have made your list, you will begin to eliminate these foods one at a time from your diet. It will take a couple of weeks before you notice any improvements. It does take some time for these foods to get through your system. However, if you do not notice any improvement, you will want to reintroduce these foods into your diet and try the next item on your list. Eventually, you will have a complete list of foods that trigger your IBS symptoms. Other popular foods to eliminate during this phase include: soy, gluten, and dairy products.

An important tool during this phase will be a food diary. This way, you will be able to keep track of which foods you are eating during the day, and any symptoms that may present themselves after they have been consumed. In general, the longer this phase is, the more likely you are to find that is triggering your IBS symptoms. It is important to remember that once eliminated, you will need to reintroduce foods slowly in the next phase.

The Reintroduction Phase

Once you have gone through your elimination period, you will be reintroducing these targeted foods back into your diet. While following the low FODMAP diet, you will need to introduce these foods back into your lifestyle one at a time.

As a tip for the reintroduction phase, we suggest starting on a Monday.

This way, you will be able to consume a small portion of the food, wait a few days, and see if you experience any symptoms. On day three, you can eat a larger portion and wait another couple days for any onset symptoms. Be sure to keep track of how you are feeling in your food diary so you can present it to a professional if need be. If you experience symptoms, this is a possible food trigger. If there is no symptom, you can assume that this certain food group is a good match for your diet.

After a while, you will have a complete list of foods that you need to assess, and you will start the elimination phase over again to double check. Once you eliminate and reintroduce, you will be able to create a diet you can stick with and eliminate any symptoms of IBS you may experience.

Maintenance Phase

While this may take time, the elimination and reintroduction phase are going to be very important while following the low FODMAP diet. These are going to be your tools in identifying foods that trigger your IBS symptom. The long-term goal is to create a wide variety of foods you can consume on a daily basis to ensure you are intaking all of your essential nutrients while eliminating the ones that make you feel lousy.

As you go through these phases, it is vital you listen to your body. Only you will be able to tell if you have a tolerance to certain foods. Remember that portion sizes will be important during these phases as well. While you may not react to small portions, larger portions may trigger the symptoms which you will want to avoid. The more tests you do, the more foods you will be able to add or subtract from your diet. While this may take some extra work, it will be worth it when you decrease your bloating and discomfort from IBS.

You may be wondering if you can follow this diet even if you have a certain lifestyle. Typically, the answer is yes! The only factor being that you could have a very limited number of foods allowed on your diet with any other limitations. Below, we will cover some of the more common diets and how you can also follow the low FODMAP diet as well!

Low FODMAP Diet with Vegan/Vegetarian Diet

If you follow a vegan or vegetarian diet, you may want to consider working with a dietary professional. Due to the fact you consume a diet that is different from most of the population, it can be more difficult to access foods that can work well with both diets. By working with a professional, they can ensure you still follow your diets without missing any essential nutrients your body needs.

While on the low FODMAP diet, it is important you keep re-testing foods. Remember that the elimination phase is meant to be short term. As you reintroduce old foods, you will be able to process if you can tolerate them or not. While you do this, you can find some staple foods, even if they happen to be high in FODMAPs.

If you follow a vegan or vegetarian diet, it will be vital that you pay special attention to your protein intake. As you will be learning later in the book, the low FODMAP diet includes a limitation of many legumes which may be a main source of protein for you right now. Instead of legumes, you can consider soy products or simply a smaller portion of legumes. Along with these switches, there are also milk substitutes to help with your protein intake. There is almond milk and other soy products to help out. Certain nuts and seeds also have varying levels of proteins for you to consider.

Low FODMAP Diet and Diabetes

If you have diabetes, you are most likely aware that there is no specific diabetic diet. In general, most people with diabetes follow a suggested balanced and healthy diet. If you wish to follow the low FODMAP diet while having diabetes, there are a few key rules you can follow to ensure you do not cause further harm to your health.

1. Planning

While on the low FODMAP diet, planning regular meals will be key. By doing this, you will be able to make sure that your blood glucose levels are always stable. By planning in advance, you can be successful in managing your diabetes while still following the low FODMAP diet. This stands especially true if you struggle finding healthy foods when you are away from your house. By being prepared, you will always have healthy options and can stay away from temptations. One good idea is to prep snacks for in-between your meals. These can be rice cakes, popcorn, or a simple fruit that is allowed in your low FODMAP diet.

2. Focus on Low FODMAP Carbohydrates

If you wish to follow the low FODMAP diet and eat healthy while having diabetes, eating starchy carbohydrates will be important for you. Some suitable options for you include wheat free bread, oats, potatoes, and rice. Before you include these, be sure to eliminate them from your diet to assure they are not triggers. Essentially, you will want to avoid any large portions of carbohydrates so you will be able to avoid any spikes in your blood glucose. You can do this by choosing slow-release carbohydrates like sweet potatoes or oats. On top of these carbs, you will also want to include allowed vegetables.

3. High Sugar Foods

As a person with diabetes, you already know that sugary foods cause your blood glucose levels to rise. On the low FODMAP diet, there is a low risk of consuming sugary foods such as soft drinks and cake, but they should still be avoided.

4. Low FODMAP Fruit

While fruits are a source of sugar, it will be important that you include a few portions of fruit per day. On the low FODMAP diet, there are plenty of options such as grapes, strawberries, bananas, and even oranges. You will want to pay special attention to your portion sizes as bigger portions, means higher amounts of fructose. You will also want to limit your portions of dried fruit, smoothies and fruit juices as they are typically pretty concentrated sources of fructose.

Low FODMAP Diet for Children

At this point, there has been very little research on the low FODMAP diet for children. Studies have shown that there are no real negative side effects for individuals who follow the low FODMAP diet for short period of time. However, if this diet were to carry on for longer than suggested, it could possibly have a negative effect on the gut flora balance in a child. If you are considering this diet for your child, there are several factors you will want to take into consideration.

First, your child will need to be seen by the pediatrician to confirm that your child has irritable bowel syndrome. Once it is diagnosed, the doctor will need to approve the diet and be carefully supervised to assure the safety of your child. Only after you follow these steps should you continue onto the elimination stage of the low FODMAP diet. For success on the diet, you can follow some of the following tips:

1. Inform Other Adults

Just like with any other diet restrictions, you will want to inform key adults of your child's restrictions. Whether it is a friend, a child care provider, or a teacher, this will be vital for the success of the diet. When these adults are in know of your child's diet, they will be able to address any stomach issues they may be having.

2. Involve Your Child

If your child is old enough, try to explain the diet to them in simple terms. You will want to explain that they are feeling sick due to the food they are eating. Be sure to include them and ask for their input in the food substitutions and menu. By making your child feel they are a part of the process, this may help your child comply with the new food rules.

3. Pack and Plan

Many parents fear diets for their children as they are always on the go! Luckily, the FODMAP diet is pretty easy to follow when you plan ahead.

When you are at home, you most likely stock the fridge with low FODMAP foods. By planning ahead and packing your own snacks and lunches, you can assure your child will stick to the diet, so they do not make themselves sick.

4. Forget the Small Stuff

Your kid is going to be a kid. If your child eats a restricted food every once in a while, it isn't going to ruin their diet altogether. Children typically do not have the self-discipline that adults have. They will most likely be tempted by restricted foods when at school or with their friends. You need to remember that while you want to stick to the diet most of the time, you can still allow your child some freedom when it comes down to what they are eating.

Exercise on the Low FODMAP Diet

While your diet may be causing your IBS symptoms, research has found that exercise can also help decrease any symptoms you may be suffering from. There are a few reasons why including regular moderate exercise will be important in the success of your diet.

First off, regular exercise can help reduce stress in your body. Typically, IBS tends to stress people out. When this happens, the nerves in your colon become tenser and can create abdominal pain. When your colon is tenser, this can slow down your bowel movements all together and cause constipation. A simple exercise such as cycling or walking can help release endorphins into your system and help release the tension in your colon. The more relaxed you are, the more flexible you will become.

Along with decreased stressed will come an increase of oxygen in your body. There are plenty of wonderful exercises such as tai chi and yoga that creates a breathing routine. When you take in these abdominal breaths, this helps increase the amount of oxygen in your body. As you increase oxygen, this will also help release any tension you are holding in your colon.

Finally, exercise can also increase your blood flow. As you begin to sweat, your body will be getting rid of toxins that could be creating discomfort in your colon. The more you sweat, the healthier you will be. Plus, the movement could help promote healthier bowel movements by moving blood to any problematic areas you may have.

As you consider exercise with your diet, remember that it will be vital to fuel your body before and after exercise. You will want to fuel about one to two hours before you work out. As long as it is included in your low FODMAP diet consider a banana with peanut butter or even oatmeal with some strawberries. The exercise can be any moderate activity of your choice from dancing, to running, to cycling, or even a little bit of strength training. Choose an exercise that makes you happy and one that you will stick with.

Reasons the Diet May Not Be Working

Speaking of sticking to a diet, some of you may follow these instructions and still suffer from IBS symptoms. If this still happens, you will want to take a look at your stress levels and the diet itself. While of course there is going to be a learning curve of the low FODMAP diet, allow yourself several weeks to change your food habits. Feel free to check back to the resources of this book to assure you are eating the foods allowed on the low FODMAP diet. If you still have no idea why you are experiencing the symptoms still, perhaps it is one of the following reasons that the diet isn't working:

1. Lack of Fiber

Fiber plays a very important role in keeping your stool regular. Often times, the low FODMAP diet will remove high fiber foods, which means you will need to pay special attention to your fiber intake. If you find yourself struggling, try speaking to a professional to find other options while on the low FODMAP diet. It will also be important that you drink plenty of water to move fiber through your system.

2. Too Much Fruit

While there are plenty of fruits on the low FODMAP diet, it is possible you are eating too much of it in one sitting. Typically, you will want to stick to only one serving at a time. If you want more fruit later in the day, try waiting two to three hours after the first one is consumed. As you practice this diet more, you will be able to tell your tolerance levels with the fruits so you can reduce that time in between servings.

3. Hidden FODMAPs

Often times, you could be consuming ingredients that are high in FODMAPs and have no idea. Typically, they are found in highly processed foods to help their taste and texture. FODMAPs are also found in some medications such as cough drops and cough syrup. Unfortunately, while they can help a cold, they are often high in sugar alcohols which can trigger your IBS symptoms. It will be important to read labels, which is included in the chapter to follow.

4. Portion Control

It is very easy to sit down and eat more than a portion. While on the low FODMAP diet, allowed foods can become high FODMAPs when you exceed their allowed portion size. As an example, you may want to enjoy some rice cakes as a treat. A recommended serving size is only two rice cakes. If you eat double the allowed portion, this is when you may experience symptoms of IBS. Again, this is where reading labels carefully will come in handy while on the low FODMAP diet.

5. Stress

Stress is going to be a huge factor on the low FODMAP diet. If you are carefully following your diet, check your lifestyle. Stress itself can cause IBS symptoms so you may want to consider stress management skills along with a diet. You can try therapy or yoga. At the end of the day, your success is in your own hands.

If you continue to have IBS symptoms after following the diet and dealing with the issues from above, you may want to seek medical advice again. It is possible you have further intolerances that have not been explored yet. Also, the FODMAP diet will not work for everyone. If you have tried and failed, ask your doctor or dietician what the next step for you could be. For now, we will begin to cover the foods you can and cannot eat while on the low FODMAP diet.

Chapter 4: Low FODMAP diet foods

In the chapter to follow, you will find a list of both low and high FODMAP foods. As for the elimination phase, you will want to try to eliminate all of the high FODMAP foods. Once you are in the reintroduction stage, you will be able to introduce these foods back in order to see what is triggering your IBS symptoms.

As you choose your foods for your low FODMAP diet, remember that reading the ingredient list on a package is going to be vital for your diet success. Below, we will cover some of the basics of reading a food label. Too often, companies are able to hide food ingredients and could be triggering your symptoms without understanding why.

When you choose your foods, portion control will also be vital. When it comes to fruit, try your best to portion out one piece every few hours. As for processed foods, you will want to avoid them all together. If you ever have any doubts on low and high FODMAP foods, you can always revisit this chapter!

Reading and Understanding Nutrition Fact Label

If you are looking to eliminate certain foods from your diet, you will be surprised to learn that they can sneak into dishes without even realizing they are there. In order to stick with your diet, learning how to read and understand a nutrition fact label is going to be crucial for your diet.

A. Serving Size

When you first look at a label, you will want to check out the serving size along with the number of servings in any given package. These serving sizes are typically standardized so you can compare them to other similar foods. Remember that for some people, they can have smaller portions of FODMAP foods, but bigger portions could trigger IBS symptoms. When you are aware of a true serving size, this will make sticking to your diet a bit easier.

B. Calories

If you are on the low FODMAP diet to lose weight, this could be helpful for you. The calories in each package provide a measurement of how much energy comes in a serving of the food. The more calories you consume, the more you will gain weight. By being mindful of the calories in a portion, you will be able to manage your weight in a healthy manner.

C. Nutrients

When you look at a label, the first ones listed are typically the ones that Americans eat a good amount of. These can include Total Fat, Saturated Fat, Trans Fat, Cholesterol, and Sodium. While this isn't the main focus of the low FODMAP diet, it is something you should be mindful of for your general health.

D. Ingredients List

Finally, you will want to pay special attention to the ingredients list included on the package. If you are intolerant to certain ingredients, you will want to keep a food journal of these foods, so you always have them at hand to compare to a label. When looking at the ingredients list, they will be listed in order of weight from most to least. Eventually, you will know exactly what you can't eat and be able to compare easily in the store. As a beginner, remember to read the label of everything you put in your shopping cart.

When you understand the basics of reading a label, it is time to move onto learning the high and low FODMAP food list. We will begin with the high FODMAP foods. With this list, you will either want to avoid the foods altogether, or reduce them drastically. Of course, everyone's tolerances will be different but to help reduce any symptoms of IBS, you should reduce the following foods to enhance your health.

High FODMAP Foods (Avoid/ Reduce)

Fruits (High Fructose)

- Apples
- Avocado
- Apricots
- Blackcurrants
- Blackberries
- Boysenberry
- Currants
- Cherries
- Dates
- Figs
- Feijoa
- Guava
- Grapefruit
- Goji Berries
- Lychee
- Mango
- Nectarines
- Prunes
- Pomegranate
- Plums
- Pineapple
- Persimmon
- Pears
- Peaches
- Raisins
- Sultana
- Tamarillo
- Watermelon

Vegetables/ Legumes

- Asparagus
- Artichoke
- Butter Beans
- Broad Beans
- Black Eyed Peas
- Beetroot
- Bananas
- Baked Beans
- Choko
- Celery

- Cauliflower
- Cassava
- Fermented Cabbage
- Garlic
- Kidney Beans
- Leek
- Lima Beans
- Mushrooms

- Mixed Vegetables
- Pickled Vegetables
- Peas
- Red Kidney Beans
- Soy Beans
- Shallots
- Scallions
- Split Peas

Cereals and Grains

- Almond Meal
- Amaranth Flour
- Breadcrumbs
- Bread
- Biscuits
- Barley
- Bran Cereals
- Crumpets
- Croissants
- Cakes
- Cashews
- Cereal Bars
- Couscous
- Egg Noodles
- Freekeh

- Gnocchi
- Muesli Cereal
- Muffins
- Pastries
- Pasta
- Pistachios
- Udon Noodles
- Wheat Bran
- Wheat Cereals
- Wheat Flour
- Wheat Germ
- Wheat Noodles
- Wheat Rolls
- Spelt Flour

Sweeteners/ Condiments

- Agave
- Fruit Bar
- Fructose
- Hummus
- Honey
- High Fructose Corn Syrup
- Jam
- Molasses
- Pesto Sauce
- Relish
- Sugar-Free Sweeteners (Inulin, Isomalt, Lactitol, Maltitol, Mannitol, Sorbitol, Xylitol)
- Tahini Paste

Drinks

- Beer
- Coconut Water
- Fruit Juices (Apple, Pear, Mango)
- Kombucha
- Malted Drink
- Quinoa Milk
- Rum
- Soy Milk
- Soda
- Tea (Black Tea, Chai Tea, Dandelion Tea, Fennel Tea, Chamomile Tea, Herbal Tea, Oolong Tea)
- Whey Protein
- Wine

Dairy

- Cheese (Cream, Halloumi, Ricotta)
- Custard

- Cream

- Ice Cream/ Gelato

- Kefir

- Milk (Cow, Goat, Evaporated Milk, Sheep)

- Sour Cream

- Yogurt

While this may seem like a large list of foods you shouldn't eat, remember that ingredients will affect individuals a little differently. While you should limit the foods listed from above, it is okay to have them every once in a while. The point of this diet is to help reduce symptoms from IBS and bloating. At the end of the day, you are in charge of what you eat and understand how certain foods will make you feel.

Low FODMAP Foods

Fruits

- Ackee
- Breadfruit
- Blueberries
- Bilberries
- Bananas (Unripe)
- Clementine
- Cranberry
- Cantaloupe
- Carambola
- Dragon Fruit
- Guava (Ripe)
- Grapes
- Honeydew
- Kiwi Fruit
- Lime
- Lemon
- Mandarin
- Orange
- Plantain
- Papaya
- Passion Fruit
- Rhubarb
- Raspberry
- Strawberry
- Tangelo
- Tamarind

Vegetables

- Alfalfa
- Butternut Squash
- Brussel Sprouts
- Broccolini
- Broccoli
- Bok Choy
- Beetroot
- Bean Sprouts
- Bamboo Shoots
- Cucumber
- Courgette
- Corn

- Choy Sum
- Cho Cho
- Chives
- Chili
- Chick Peas
- Celery
- Carrots
- Cabbage
- Eggplant
- Fennel
- Ginger
- Green Pepper
- Green Beans
- Kale
- Leek Leaves
- Lentils
- Lettuce
- Olives
- Okra

- Pumpkin
- Peas (Snow)
- Parsnip
- Red Peppers
- Radish
- Sweet Potato
- Swiss Chard
- Sun-Dried Tomatoes
- Squash
- Spinach
- Spaghetti Squash
- Seaweed
- Scallions
- Turnip
- Tomato
- Water Chestnuts
- Yams
- Zucchin

Meat and Poultry

- Beef
- Chicken
- Deli Meats
- Lamb

- Prosciutto
- Pork
- Turkey
- Processed Meats

Seafood and Fish

- **Fresh Fish (Cod, Haddock, Salmon, Trout, Tuna, Canned Tuna)**
- **Seafood (Crab, Lobster, Mussels, Oysters, Shrimp)**

Breads, Cereals, Grains, and Nuts

- Bread
  Wheat Free
  Gluten Free
  Potato Flour
  Spelt Sourdough
  Rice
  Oat
  Corn
- Pasta
  Wheat Free
  Gluten Free
- Almonds
- Biscuit (Shortbread)
- Buckwheat (Noodles, Flour)
- Brazil Nuts
- Brown Rice
- Crackers
- Corn Tortillas
- Coconut Milk
- Cornflakes
- Corncakes
- Crispbread
- Corn Flour
- Chips (Plain)
- Mixed Nuts
- Millet
- Macadamia Nuts
- Oatcakes
- Oats
- Oatmeal
- Pretzels
- Potato Flour
- Popcorn
- Polenta

- Pine Nuts
- Pecans
- Rice
    White
    Rice
    Brown
    Basmati
- Rice Krispies
- Rice Flour
- Rice Crackers

- Rice Cakes
- Rice Bran
- Seeds
    Sunflower
    Sesame
    Pumpkin
    Poppy
    Chai
- Tortilla Chips
- Walnuts

Condiments, Sweets, and Sweeteners

- Almond Butter
- Acesulfame K
- Aspartame
- Chocolate
    White
    Milk
    Dark
- Erythritol
- Fish Sauce
- Glycerol
- Glucose
- Golden Syrup
- Jelly

- Ketchup
- Mustard
- Miso Paste
- Mayonnaise
- Marmite
- Marmalade
- Maple Syrup
- Oyster Sauce
- Peanut Butter
- Rice Malt Syrup
- Sucralose (Sugar)
- Stevia

- Sweet and Sour Sauce
- Shrimp Paste
- Saccharine
- Tomato Sauce
- Tamarind

- Vinegar
  - Rice Wine Vinegar
  - Balsamic Vinegar
  - Apple Cider Vinegar
- Worcestershire Sauce
- Wasabi

Drinks

- Alcohol (Wine, Whiskey, Gin, Vodka, Beer)
- Coffee
- Chocolate Powder
- Protein Powder (Whey,

  Rice, Pea, Egg)
- Soya Milk
- Sugar-Free Soft Drinks
- Water

Dairy/ Eggs

- Butter
- Cheese (Swiss, Ricotta, Parmesan, Mozzarella, Goat, Fetta, Cottage, Cheddar, Camembert, Brie)
- Eggs
- Milk (Rice, Oat, Macadamia, Lactose-free,

  Hemp, Almond)
- Swiss Cheese
- Soy Protein
- Sorbet
- Tofu
- Tempeh
- Yogurt (Goat, Lactose-free, Greek, Coconut)

Herbs and Spices

- Bay Leaves
- Basil
- Curry Leaves
- Coriander
- Cilantro
- Fenugreek
- Lemongrass
- Mint
- Oregano
- Parsley
- Rosemary
- Sage
- Thyme
- Tarragon
- All Spice
- Black Pepper
- Chili Powder
- Cardamom
- Curry Powder
- Cumin
- Cloves
- Five Spice
- Fennel Seeds

- Nutmeg
- Saffron
- Turmeric
- Avocado Oil
- Coconut Oil
- Canola Oil
- Olive Oil
- Sesame Oil
- Sunflower Oil
- Soy Bean Oil
- Vegetable Oil
- Baking Soda
- Baking Powder
- Cocoa Powder
- Ghee
- Gelatin
- Lard
- Salt
- Yeast

As you can tell from the list from above, there are food choices for all different types of diets. Whether you are vegan, vegetarian, or follow a typical diet, there are plenty of choices for you.

The list from above may seem daunting, but as you learn your own version of the low FODMAP diet, you will be able to put together recipes from the ingredients you are allowed. The key to being successful on this diet is enjoying the foods you are allowed. Luckily in today's market, there are plenty of substitutes for ingredients that may trigger you. As long as you take the time to make this list, you will be able to make your new diet successful.

In the chapter to follow, we will be providing a couple different meal plans for you to follow. There will be a seven-day example vegan diet. Once you have read through this, you can move onto the fourteen-day low FODMAP starter diet. Remember that these are mere suggestions and you can make adjustments as needed.

Chapter 5: Low FODMAP Diet Meal plan

At this point in the book, you hopefully have a better understanding of the foods you can and cannot eat while on the low FODMAP diet. Before we jump into potential meal plans for you to follow, it is time to learn some delicious ingredients.

If you feel nervous about the diet due to the big list of foods to avoid, you absolutely shouldn't! Is your diet going to be different? Yes. However, when you are no longer experiencing diarrhea, constipation, bloating, and the other symptoms from IBS, you will be asking yourself why you didn't start sooner!

As you will find out from the recipes from below, there is a way to stick to your diet and enjoy your meal at the same time. You will find easy to make breakfast, lunch, and dinner recipes. Remember to pay special attention to the ingredients so you can determine if the recipe itself will stick within your own limits.

Low FODMAP Breakfast Recipes:

Small Banana Pancakes

Prep Time: Five Minutes

Cook Time: Twenty Minutes

Servings: Two

Portion: Four Mini Pancakes

Ingredients:

- Dairy-free Spread (Olive Oil) (3 T.)
- Ground Nutmeg (.25 t.)
- Ground Cinnamon (.50 t.)
- Salt (.125 t.)
- Baking Powder (.25 t.)
- Brown Sugar (1 T.)
- Gluten-free All-Purpose Flour (2 T.)
- Egg (2)
- Banana (2 Small, Unripe)

Instructions

1. Begin by heating a medium pan over medium heat before tossing in your dairy-free spread.
2. While this is cooking, go ahead and peel the banana before placing it into a bowl. Mash the banana until it becomes smooth and then add in the egg.
3. Once the egg and banana are mixed well, go ahead and add in the rest of the ingredients. At this point, you should have a mixture that resembles batter.
4. Spoon the mixture into your heated pan and cook the pancakes for a few minutes on each side or until they turn a nice golden color.
5. For extra flavor, try topping the pancakes with your favorite low FODMAP fruit!

Roasted Sausage and Vegetable Breakfast Casserole

Prep Time: Twenty-Five Minutes

Cook Time: Forty-Five Minutes

Servings: Eight

Ingredients:

- Eggs (12)
- Low FODMAP Milk (.50 C.)
- Dried Oregano (.50 t.)
- Salt and Pepper (.25 t.)
- Leek Tips (.50 C.)
- Red Bell Pepper (1)
- Lamb Sausage (1 Package)
- Baby Spinach (2 C.)
- Potato (1)
- Butternut Squash (1)
- Sweet Potato (1)
- Olive Oil (1 T.)

Instructions:

1. Before you begin prepping your food, you will want to preheat your oven to 400 degrees.
2. As your oven heats up, prepare the vegetables from the list above by peeling them and dicing the ingredients into bite-size pieces.

3. Once this is done, place the vegetables on a tray and drizzle them lightly with olive oil or a spread that is allowed on your own low FODMAP diet. Pop them into the heated oven for twenty minutes or until they are soft.

4. While the vegetables are cooking, you can cook your red bell pepper, leek, and sausage in a pan over medium heat. Be sure to cook all of these ingredients through.

5. Now that all of these ingredients are cooked, add in the vegetables to a large casserole dish.

6. In a small bowl, mix together the eggs and add in desired spices. When ready, gently pour the mix over the vegetables already placed in the casserole dish.

7. Place the dish in the oven for thirty minutes or until the eggs are set. This is a great dish to enjoy hot or cold for breakfast!

Blueberry Low FODMAP Smoothie

Prep Time: Five Minutes

Servings: One

Ingredients:

- Lemon Juice (1 t.)
- Maple Syrup (.50 T.)
- Rice Protein Powder (2 t.)
- Frozen Banana (1)
- Ice Cubes (6-10)
- Blueberries (20)
- Vanilla Soy Ice cream (.25 C.)
- Low FODMAP Milk (.50 C.)

Instructions:

1. Place all of the ingredients from above into a blender. Be sure to cut the frozen banana into smaller pieces.
2. Serve right away for a delicious breakfast.

Banana and Oats FODMAP Breakfast Smoothie

Prep Time: Five Minutes

Servings: One

Ingredients:

- Almond Milk (.50 C.)
- Linseeds (1 t.)
- Rolled Oats (1 T.)
- Banana (1)

Instructions:

1. Place all of the ingredients from above into a blender. Be sure you cut the banana into smaller pieces for easier blending.
2. Serve immediately for a filling and healthy meal.

Blueberry, Banana, and Peanut Butter Breakfast Smoothie

Prep Time: Five Minutes

Servings: One

Ingredients:

- Ice Cubes (6-10)
- Low FODMAP Milk (.75 C.)
- Blueberries (.50 C.)
- Peanut Butter (1 T.)
- Banana (.50)

Instructions:

1. Place all of the ingredients from above into a blender and blend until everything is smooth.
2. Serve immediately and enjoy!

Kale, Ginger, and Pineapple Breakfast Smoothie

Prep Time: Five Minutes

Servings: One

Ingredients:

- Ice (1 C.)
- Ginger (.25 T.)
- Kale (1 C.)
- Pineapple (.75 C.)
- Orange (.50)
- Low FODMAP Milk (1 C.)

Instructions:

1. Place all of the ingredients from above into a blender and blend until everything becomes smooth.
2. Serve immediately for a nice, healthy breakfast.

Strawberry and Banana Breakfast Smoothie

Prep: Five Minutes

Servings: One

Ingredients:

- Ice (1 C.)
- Maple Syrup (1 t.)
- Low FODMAP Milk (.75 C.)
- Strawberries (6)
- Banana (1)

Instructions:

1. Toss all of the ingredients into your blender and mix together until smooth.
2. Serve and for an extra treat, try adding some whipped cream!

Low FODMAP Soups and Salads:

Apple, Carrot, and Kale Salad

Prep Time: Ten Minute

Servings: Eight

Portion: .50 C.

Ingredients:

- Salt and Pepper (.25 t.)
- Maple Syrup (1.50 t.)
- Mustard (1 T.)
- Red Wine Vinegar (1.50 T.)
- Olive Oil (3 T.)
- Kale (.50 C.)
- Carrots (3)
- Apple (1 C.)

Instructions:

1. First step, you will want to create your dressing for the salad. You can do this by taking a small bowl and mixing together the maple syrup, mustard, vinegar, and oil. For some extra flavor, season with salt and pepper to taste.

2. Once this is done, take the kale, carrots, and apple and chop into fine, smaller pieces.

3. Finally, dress the salad, toss it a bit, and your meal is ready to be served!

Green Bean, Tomato, and Chicken Salad

Prep Time: Fifteen Minutes

Servings: Four

Portion: .50 C.

Ingredients:

- Lettuce (1 C.)
- Basil Leaves (2 T.)
- Cherry Tomatoes (10)
- Gruyere Cheese (.50 C.)
- Cooked Chicken (1 Lb.)
- Green Beans (.50 C.)

Instructions:

1. To begin, you will want to bring a medium pot of water to a boil. Once the water is boiling, cook your green beans for a few minutes. Once they are tender, drain the water from the pot and run the beans under cold water for a minute.
2. Next, take a large bowl and mix together all of the ingredients from above for a healthy salad.
3. For extra flavor, top your salad with any low FODMAP approved dressings.

Tuna Salad Low FODMAP Style

Prep Time: Five Minutes

Servings: Six

Portion: .50 C.

Ingredients:

- Salt and Pepper (to taste)
- Dried Dill (.50 t.)
- Lemon Juice (1.50 T.)
- Mayonnaise (.50 C.)
- Celery (.50)
- Tuna (2 Cans)

Instructions:

1. Start out by squeezing the liquid out of the tuna.
2. Once you have discarded the tuna, add it into a medium bowl with the vegetables from above.
3. When everything is stirred together, add in the dill, lemon juice, mayonnaise, along with the salt and pepper.
4. This mixture is great for any salad or sandwich!

Low FODMAP Pumpkin Soup

Prep Time: Ten Minutes

Cook Time: Fifteen Minutes

Servings: Six

Portion: 1 C.

Ingredients:

- Lactose-free Half and Half (.75 C.)
- Light Brown Sugar (1 T.)
- Canned Pure Pumpkin (1)
- Vegetable Soup Base (2 T.)
- Water (3 C.)
- Cayenne Pepper (.125 t.)
- Nutmeg (.25 t.)
- Cinnamon (.25 t.)
- Smoked Paprika (.25 t.)
- Scallions (.75 C.)
- Olive Oil (1 T.)
- Unsalted Butter (2 T.)
- Salt and Pepper to taste

Instructions:

1. To begin, you will want to heat up a medium sized pot over a low to medium heat. Once the pot is warm, you can add in your oil and butter until it begins to sizzle.

2. When the butter and oil are warm, add in your spices with the scallions and cook until they are soft.

3. Once this happens, add in the soup and water. Be sure to mix everything together before you add in the salt, brown sugar, and the canned pumpkin.

4. Now that these ingredients are placed in the pot, lower your heat and allow these to simmer for ten minutes or so. Feel free to stir every once in a while, to assure the ingredients are blended well.

5. Now, remove the soup from the heat and add in your half and half. Once the soup is cool, you can place the mixture into a blender and blend until it is smooth.

6. For extra flavor, season the soup with salt and pepper to taste.

Quinoa and Turkey Meatball Soup

Prep Time: Fifteen Minutes

Cook Time: Twenty Minutes

Servings: Eight

Portion: 1 C.

Ingredients:

- Collard Greens (5 C.)
- Celery (.50)
- Leek Tips (1 C.)
- Olive Oil (2 T.)
- Egg (1)
- Dried Basil (2 T.)
- Parsley (2 T.)
- Cooked Quinoa (.50 C.)
- Ground Turkey (1 Lb.)
- Turkey Stock (10 C.)
- Salt and Pepper to taste

Instructions:

1. To start out, you are going to want to make your meatballs for the soup. You will do this by taking a large mixing bowl and combine the egg, parsley, basil, quinoa, and turkey together.

Gently take the mixture in your hands and form one inch balls.

2. Next, take a medium pan over medium heat and cook the turkey meatballs in olive oil for a few minutes. Be sure to flip the balls over so that they are a nice golden-brown color all around.

3. Now that these are done, take a large pot over medium heat and add in a tablespoon of oil. Once the oil is sizzling, you can add in the leek and celery. Sauté these two ingredients for a minute before adding in the collard greens and stock.

4. When all of the ingredients are cooked, add in the meatballs and allow this mixture to simmer over a low heat for eight to ten minutes.

5. Remove the soup from the heat and allow to cool slightly before serving.

Mixed Vegetable, Bean and Pasta Soup

Prep Time: Fifteen Minutes

Cook Time: Thirty Minutes

Servings: Fourteen

Portion: .75 C.

Ingredients:

- Gluten-free Pasta (1 C.)
- Dried Thyme (1 t.)
- Smoked Paprika (1 t.)
- Dried Basil (1 t.)
- Zucchini (1)
- Squash (1)
- Bok Choy (2 C.)
- Carrots (3)
- Kale (1 C.)
- Red Potatoes (1 C.)
- Butternut Squash (1 C.)
- Crushed Tomatoes (1 Can)
- Water (8 C.)
- Leek Tips (.25 C.)
- Scallions (.75 C.)
- Olive Oil (2 T.)
- Salt and Pepper to taste

Instructions:

1. To start, you will want to take a large pot and begin to heat it over medium heat with the olive oil placed in the bottom.

2. Once the olive oil is sizzling, add in the leeks and scallions and allow them to cook until they become soft.

3. When these are ready, add in your prepared zucchini, squash, Bok choy, carrots, kale, potatoes, chickpeas, canned tomatoes, and the water. Season as desired and place the top on the pot.

4. Bring all of the ingredients from above to a boil and then turn the heat down to allow everything to simmer for at least thirty minutes. By the end, all of the vegetables should be tender.

5. While the soup cooks, you can cook the gluten-free pasta in another pot so by the end, you can combine everything and have a healthy meal!

Vegan Options:

Low FODMAP Coconut and Banana Breakfast Cookie

Prep Time: Ten Minutes

Cook Time: Twenty Minutes

Servings: Ten

Portion: One

Ingredients:

- Vanilla Extract (1 t.)
- Vegetable Oil (.25 C.)
- Maple Syrup (.25 C.)
- Banana (1)
- Baking Powder (.50 t.)
- Cinnamon (1 t.)
- Ground Flax Seeds (2 T.)
- Chia Seeds (2 T.)
- Unsweetened Coconut Flakes (.50 C.)
- Banana Chips (.50 C.)
- Gluten-free All-purpose Flour (.50 C.)
- Old-fashioned Oats (1 C.)

Instructions:

1. You will want to begin by heating your oven to 325 degrees.

2. While the oven heats up, take a medium bowl and mix together the baking powder, cinnamon, flax seeds, chia seeds, coconut flakes, banana chips, flour, and oats altogether.

3. In another bowl, mix together a mashed banana, vanilla, vegetable oil, and pale syrup. When both bowls are well combined, you can mix them together and begin to create your dough.

4. Next, take a greased cookie sheet and lay out balls of dough to create your cookies. When this is done, pop the cookie sheet in the oven for twenty minutes.

5. When the time is up, remove the cookies, allow to cool, and enjoy!

Lemon and Garlic Roasted Zucchini

Prep Time: Five Minutes

Cook Time: Twenty Minutes

Servings: Twelve

Portion: 1 C.

Ingredients:

- Olive Oil (1.50 T.)
- Zucchini (2)
- Lemon Zest (2 T.)
- Salt and Pepper to taste

Instructions:

1. You can begin by heating your oven to 425 degrees.
2. While this warms up, slice your zucchini into thin slices and place in a bowl with the lemon zest and olive oil. Assure it is covered completely before seasoning with salt and pepper.
3. Place the zucchini on a greased sheet pan and cook for twenty minutes.

Rainbow Low FODMAP Slaw

Prep Time: Ten Minutes

Servings: Twenty

Portion: 1 C.

Ingredients:

- Pomegranate Seeds (.50 C.)
- Carrots (3)
- Kale (1 C.)
- Red Cabbage (1 C.)
- Green Cabbage (1 C.)
- Lactose-free Yogurt (.50 C.)
- Dijon Mustard (1 t.)
- Sugar (2 T.)
- Apple Cider Vinegar (.25 C.)
- Canola Oil (.50 C.)

Ingredients:

1. Start out by creating your dressing for the slaw. You can do this in a small bowl, mix together the canola oil, apple cider vinegar, Dijon mustard, sugar, yogurt, and a little bit of salt.
2. In another bowl, toss together the different cabbage with the carrots and the kale.
3. Gently drizzle the dressing over the kale, and you have a delicious slaw that is full of color and flavor!

Vegan Roasted Red Pepper Farfalle

Prep Time: Ten Minutes

Cook Time: Ten Minutes

Servings: Four

Portion: 1 C.

Ingredients:

- Capers (.25 C.)
- Parsley (.75 C.)
- Olive Oil (.25 C.)
- Roasted Red Peppers (1 Jar)
- Gluten-free Farfalle Pasta (2 C.)

Instructions:

1. You can start this recipe by cooking your pasta according to the instructions on the side of the box.
2. Once the pasta is cooked through, drain the water and then place the pasta back into the pot.
3. Toss in the oil, parsley, roasted red peppers, and capers to the mixture.
4. Mix everything together and season with salt and pepper for extra flavor.

As you can tell, you can follow the low FODMAP diet and still enjoy delicious foods. While these are only some of the many recipes you can follow on your diet, there are plenty of resources out there to provide you with even more! With these resources in hand, we will now go over a simple seven and fourteen-day meal plan that is easy to follow.

With a limited food choices, you may be thinking to yourself that you are going to get bored quick. When it comes to a new diet, it is all about your frame of mind. On one hand, you could think negatively about it and return to your old eating habits. With choice, comes consequence. When you eat the foods that trigger you, you are going to feel lousy. Why make that choice when you can choose to eat healthy and feel better? Below, we will provide some simple meals for you to consider until you feel confident enough to create your own recipes

Breakfast Meal Plan Ideas:

- Eggs- Hard-boiled, over easy, or even scrambled. There are many ways to enjoy eggs!
- Lactose-Free Yogurt with any low FODMAP fruit
- Gluten-free Muffins
- Gluten-free French toast
- Gluten-free Oatmeal with cinnamon
- Rice Cereal with low FODMAP fruit
- Ground Turkey
- Smoothie with low FODMAP fruit

Lunch Meal Plan Ideas:

- Gluten-free Bread with Deli Meat and Cheese
- Chicken Noodle Soup
- Quinoa Bowl with low FODMAP Veggies or Grilled Chicken
- Salad
- Baked Potato with Lactose-free Butter

Dinner Meal Plan Ideas:

- Stir-Fried Rice
- Tacos
- Gluten-Free Pizza
- Grilled Chicken Salad
- Steak with Fresh Low FODMAP Vegetables
- Grilled Chicken with White Rice
- Rice Pasta with Marinara
- Snack Meal Plan Ideas:
- Rice Cakes with Peanut Butter
- Baby Carrots
- Lactose-free Yogurt
- Unripe Banana
- Unsalted Peanuts
- Pop Chips
- Gluten-free Pretzels
- Crackers with Cheese
- Hard-Boiled Egg

14- Day Meal Plan

Week One:

Meal	Monday	Tues.	Wed.	Thurs.	Friday
BFast	Small Banana Pancakes	Blueberry Smoothie	Roasted Sausage and Vegetable Breakfast Casserole	Strawberry and Banana Breakfast Smoothie	Banana and Oats FODMAP Breakfast Smoothie
Lunch	Apple, Carrot, and Kale Salad	Mixed Vegetable, Bean, and Pasta Soup	Low FODMAP Pumpkin Soup	Tuna Salad Low FODMAP Style	Quinoa and Turkey Meatball Soup
Dinner	Low FODMAP Veggie Latkes	Steak with Lemon and Garlic Roasted Zucchini	Left Over Mixed Vegetable, Bean, and Pasta Soup	Vegan Roasted Red Pepper Farfalle	Salad with Grilled Chicken and Homemade Dressing

Meal	Saturday	Sunday
Breakfast	Eggs and low FODMAP fruit	Rice Cereal with low FODMAP fruit
Lunch	Chicken Noodle Soup	Baked Potato with Lactose-free Butter
Dinner	Stir-Fried Rice	Gluten-free Pizza

Week Two:

Meal	Monday	Tuesday	Wednesday	Thursday	Friday
Breakfast	Gluten-free French Toast	Rice Cereal with low FODMAP fruit	Lactose-free Yogurt with low FODMAP fruit	Blueberry Smoothie	Small Banana Pancakes
Lunch	Quinoa Bowl	Salad with Approved Dressing	Gluten-free Sandwich with Deli Meat and Cheese	Mixed Vegetable, Bean, and Pasta Soup	Tuna Salad on Gluten-free Bread
Dinner	Grilled Chicken with White Rice	Grilled Chicken Salad	Salad with Approved Dressing	Gluten-free Tacos	Stir-Fried Rice

Meal	Saturday	Sunday
Breakfast	Smoothie with low FODMAP fruit	Lactose-free Yogurt with low FODMAP fruit
Lunch	Rice Pasta with Marinara	Chicken Noodle Soup
Dinner	Baked Potato with Lactose-free Butter	Grilled Chicken Salad

Vegan 7-Day Meal Plan

Meal	Monday	Tuesday	Wednesday	Thursday	Friday
Breakfast	Coconut Yogurt with Chia Seeds	Rice Cakes with Peanut Butter	Corn Flakes with Almond Milk	Gluten-free Bread with Almond Butter	Unripe Banana with Coconut Yogurt
Lunch	Lemon and Garlic Roasted Zucchini	Rainbow Low FODMAP Slaw with Gluten-free Bread	Vegan Roasted Red Pepper Farfalle	Low FODMAP Coconut and Banana Cookie with Coconut Yogurt	Salad with Approved Dressing
Dinner	Low FODMAP Veggie Latkes	Gluten-free Pasta with Approved Sauce	Plain Tempeh with low FODMAP Veggie of choice	Plain Tofu with Rice Noodles	Gluten-free Pizza with Soy Cheese

Meal	Saturday	Sunday
Breakfast	Blueberry Smoothie with Coconut Milk	Banana and Oat Smoothie with Coconut Milk
Lunch	Plain Tofu with Soba Noodles	Plain Tempeh with Gluten-free Pasta
Dinner	Grilled Cabbage Soup	Baked Brussel Sprouts with Plain Tofu

Chapter 6: Low FODMAP diet tips and tricks for success

Starting a new diet can be scary. As we said before, your frame of mind is going to be incredibly important. It is vital you think about your why when making food choices. Each meal, we have a chance to better our health; all it takes is a little thought behind each decision.

Of course, we want to see you succeed with your diet. Below, you will find a number of tips and tricks that have helped other clients on the low FODMAP diet. While some may work for you, others may not. You must adjust the low FODMAP diet to match your desired lifestyle so you not only stick with it but can enjoy it at the same time!

1. Read the Label

Reading the labels on packaged foods is going to be vital for the success of your diet. Unfortunately, many high FODMAP ingredients can have very confusing names. We suggest carrying a list of additives to avoid until you learn them by heart. When you are more aware, you can avoid the high FODMAP ingredients.

2. Water-soluble

In general, low FODMAP foods are going to be water-soluble, but this does not mean they are fat-soluble. If you are cooking a soup with an onion, you will want to take the onion out. Instead, try using onion-infused oils for the taste. It is quick fix that may help with your IBS triggers.

1. High Fructose Corn Syrup

High Fructose Corn Syrup is in everything. Again, it will be important that you learn how to read food labels so you will be able to avoid this mistake. This ingredient is in a number of foods including energy bars, juices, mayonnaise, frozen meals, and even popcorn. Check the label before you put anything into your shopping cart.

2. Fiber

If you pick up a product and it seems to have a high serving f fiber, you can assume it is due to a high FODMAP additive. Try to avoid any products that boast about their fiber; it's a trap! Any fiber additives will more than likely trigger your GI issues.

3. Onion and Garlic Powder

When it comes to choosing out your spices, pay special attention to the labels. You will want to avoid onion and garlic powders as they contain high FODMAPs. Luckily, there are plenty of delicious low FODMAP approved spices as you can find in the chapter from above.

4. "Natural"

If you find any frozen foods, brothers, or savory soups that claim they have "natural" flavors, go ahead and check out the label. You can assume that they contain garlic and onion, very popular IBS triggers. You will want to try your best to avoid these additives to your meals.

5. "Healthy"

As much as we would like to trust when products claim they are healthy, this does not equate to low FODMAP approved. Foods like asparagus and apples are supposedly "healthy" for you, but they can trigger IBS symptoms. As you go through the elimination process, you will learn just what you can and cannot eat and make the decision if something is healthy for you.

6. Beverages

Often times, people forget that beverages can contain FODMAPs. You will want to pay special attention to what you are putting into your body. If you ever have questions, feel free to refer to our lists in the chapter from above. Just because a beverage claims it has no net carbohydrates, this does not mean they aren't high in FODMAPs.

7. Portion Control

While you are on the low FODMAP diet, portion is going to be key to success. When you are reading labels, you will always want to pay special attention to portion size. While a low FODMAP diet is approved, a bigger portion may still trigger IBS symptoms. You will want to try your best to be mindful of portion control.

8. Learn About Yourself

As you start this diet, you will want to spend plenty of time on the elimination phase. The more you test, the more you will be able to figure out what foods you can and cannot eat. When you have more to choose from, you will be able to get more creative with your recipes. At the end of the day, only you know what is best for you. When you learn yourself, the diet will become that much easier.

9. Food and Meal Journal

Your food and meal journal are going to be an important tool for your low FODMAP diet journey. By keeping track of the foods, you can and cannot eat; it will make it easier when you go back to check out your history. We eat so many different types of foods through the day; it can be hard to remember which foods trigger you. By keeping a journal, it leaves little room for mistakes.

10. Use Your Fridge

If you are trying your best to stick with the low FODMAP diet, why leave anything up to chance? Do yourself a favor and take the time to remove any high FODMAP foods in your house. By keeping your pantry and fridge stocked with the low FODMAP foods you need, it deletes any temptations you may have in the house.

11. Have A Backup Plan

Dieting is hard, especially when you are first starting out. When you are planning out your meals, it is possible to miss one here or there. Try to stack your freezer with low FODMAP meals so you can cook them in a few minutes. When your first plan falls through, you will always have a backup. It is a win-win situation!

Chapter 7: Low FODMAP diet FAQ

As we are nearing our time together, hopefully, you are feeling better about starting the low FODMAP diet. While you have learned a lot about the diet, feel free to check back whenever you have a question about the diet. Whether you need a refresher on the benefits of the diet or a reminder of which foods you can and cannot eat, you will be able to find the information here easily.

To finish off, we will hopefully be able to answer any further questions you have about the low FODMAP diet. Simply remember that this diet is going to be specifically tailored up to you. Being diagnosed with IBS or other GI tract issues is not the end of the world. It will take some extra effort, but when your symptoms and discomfort are relieved, you will be thankful you made the choice to start the low FODMAP diet. For now, it is time to answer some more popular questions you may still have.

Q. I am following the low FODMAP diet and still experiencing symptoms, is this the right diet for me?

A. The answer could be yes and no. If you are following the diet and still find yourself with symptoms of IBS, there may be another culprit in your diet. Remember to keep a food diet with you at all times so you can find any triggers you may be missing.

Q. Can I follow the low FODMAP diet as a vegetarian?

A. Absolutely! You can follow this diet whether you are vegan or vegetarian, it will just take a little extra work. You will find in the chapters before there are plenty of choices, so long as the allowed foods are not triggers for your own body. Some good sources of protein for this diet would be chickpeas, tofu, tempeh, and more. If there is a will, there is always a way!

Q. How do I make sure I'm getting enough Fiber?

A. This is one of the bigger concerns for those following the low FODMAP diet, especially if constipation is an issue. Luckily, several good low FODMAP sources can help you keep your fiber intake up. These include chia seeds, brown rice, flax seeds, kiwi, oranges, white potato, rice bran and more. Check out the list provided in the fourth chapter for a longer list.

Q. Should I eat Larger or Smaller Meals on the Low FODMAP Diet?

A. In general, you should try to eat three main meals through your day and to snacks between these meals. If you are still hungry, you can always add in another snack. Remember that portion control is going to be vital while you are on the low FODMAP diet, so this is something you will want to keep in mind when plating your meals.

Q. What is the rule with fats and oils on the Low FODMAP Diet?

A. As a general rule, there are plenty of fats and oils that are low in FODMAPs. However, anything in excess can trigger IBS symptoms. You will want to be especially aware of any condiments or sauces that are oil-based such as salad dressings. Most of the time, these also include high FODMAPs like garlic. Remember to always read the labels before consuming anything. You can also refer to our extended grocery list to see which fats and oils are allowed on the diet.

Q. Can I eat meat on the low FODMAP Diet?

A. Yes and No. Some sources of animal protein such as fish and chicken are low in FODMAPs. However, if the meat is prepared already, you will want to avoid any additives that may trigger your symptoms. If you have any further questions, please refer to the food lists from the chapter above.

Q. What happens if I break my diet?

A. While the aim of the diet is to stick to it as much as possible, mistakes and slip ups will happen. Overall, you will want to achieve control over any symptoms you may be having. If you slip up, expect to experience the IBS symptoms. As long as you return to your diet, you will most likely be able to improve them in a few days.

Q. Is this a lifestyle?

A. No, the low FODMAP diet is not meant to last for a lifetime. The aim of the diet is to help heal your gut over a controlled period of time. This diet should only be followed for two to six weeks. After this, you can begin to introduce food back into your diet. This will change depending on each individual.

PART 2

Chapter 1: What is The Freestyle Way?

As you begin your journey using the Freestyle techniques, you will learn it utilizes the elements of calories in and calories out. The point system assigns specific points based on the nutritional and calorie content. Your activity level also influences how the points are assigned to offset against the food points.

One excellent online resource to discover your points is available at "healthyweightforum.org/eng/calculators/ww-points-allowed/" The information involved includes your gender, age, activity level, weight, height, and how many pounds you want to lose. The math is calculated for you to show how many points you can consume on your meal plan daily.

For example, a 65-year old woman who has a sedentary lifestyle, is 5'1" tall, 174 lbs. who wants to lose 10 pounds is allowed 24 points for the first 2 weeks and 23 points for the next 3 weeks.

All you need to do is add the points for additional optional or toppings that are not included in the recipe. Each food added to the product will possibly raise the content of fat or sugar. Proteins are calculated into the equation to help lower the points.

The goal is to get you on the right track of choosing leaner proteins and eating more fruits and vegetables with each meal. By increasing these food items, you are lowering the unhealthy fats and consuming less sugar. You will be surprised by many of the foods that contain -0- points. It's hard to believe they are diet-friendly foods!

Use your enclosed 21-day plan as a guideline to get your body in tune with the new way of eating healthier. It won't take long before you are inspired. Your family and friends will surely enjoy the tastier techniques used for food preparation. You will also love all of the new zero foods!

Zero Point Fruits

Enjoy most fruits in moderation - only because the calories can add up quickly. The only exceptions to the rule are plantains and avocados. Consider this as you prepare your smoothie, if you add any additional fruits - be sure to consider any possible points involved. This includes frozen or fresh fruit, as well as jarred or canned. Just remember to choose the ones packaged without added sugar.

Zero Point Vegetables

Many veggies are -0- points on the new Freestyle plan. However, as you prepare your meal, be sure to take into accounts the oil and butter used as you make the vegetables. Enjoy canned, fresh or frozen mushy peas, potatoes, parsnips, cassava, yuca, yams, sweet potatoes, and olives - without additional fats, oil, or sugars.

Zero Point Spices & Other Condiments

You can choose from many items including low-sugar condiments and spices. For example, enjoy items such as fresh or rubs, vinegar, broth, dried spices, hot sauce, mustard, salsa, and capers.

Remember, the points consumed will also depend on the amount you are using in your recipe. They may be zero points for a small serving, but collectively, as they are used in the recipe, they may contain more points.

Other Foods To Enjoy Freestyle

- Boneless & skinless chicken breast and turkey

- Ground lean chicken and turkey

- Thinly sliced deli chicken or turkey breast

- All shellfish and fish (excluding smoked or dried fish)

- Canned fish packed in brine or water

- Regular and smoked tofu

- Eggs

- Plain soy yogurt

- Plain Greek yogurt

- Fresh – frozen - canned beans and lentils that are packed without oil or sugar (Ex. Lentils, pinto beans, split peas, chickpeas, black beans, kidney beans, soybeans, and more)

Chapter 2: Breakfast Favorites

No matter what you are craving, just remember, breakfast is considered the most important meal of the day. So, enjoy each one of these selections as you adjust to your new way of meal preparation!

Baked Omelet

Freestyle Points: 2

Yields: 4 Servings

Ingredients:

- Egg whites – 3
- Large eggs - 3
- Greek yogurt - plain fat-free – 2 tbsp.
- Pepper - .25 tsp.
- Salt - .125 tsp.
- Onion - .25 cup
- Bell peppers - .25 cup
- Grated parmesan cheese - .25 cup
- Cubed ham - .5 cup
- Broccoli florets – 1 cup
- Baby spinach leaves – 2 cups
- For the Garnish: Green onion – 1
- Also Needed:
- -10-inch skillet

Preparation Method:

1. Warm up the temperature setting in the oven to 400°F.

2. Chop the veggies. Whip the yogurt, eggs, pepper, and salt until frothy using a hand mixer.

3. Warm up the skillet using the med-high setting and spray with oil to prevent sticking. Add the broccoli, peppers, ham, and onions. Lower the temperature to the medium heat setting. Continue cooking for approximately five minutes.

4. Toss in the spinach and continue cooking until wilted. Blend in the green onions and add the mixed eggs. Sprinkle with the parmesan.

5. Cook 10 minutes on the stovetop. Move it to the oven for 10 to 15 additional minutes until the eggs are done and set.

6. Garnish with a few green onions and parmesan cheese before serving.

Banana Roll-Ups

Freestyle Points:2

Yields: 1 Serving

Ingredients:

- Whole wheat bread – low-cal – 1 slice
- Medium peeled banana - .5 of 1
- Salt-free chunky peanut butter - 1.5 tsp.

Preparation Method:

1. Use a rolling pin or wine bottle as a substitute to flatten the bread.
2. Apply the peanut butter to one side of the bread. Add the banana.
3. Roll it up and slice into 3-4 segments.
4. Enjoy any time.

Broccoli Cheddar Egg Muffins

Freestyle Points: 2

Yields: 6 Servings

Ingredients:

- Egg whites - 4
- Whole eggs- 8
- Dijon mustard -.5 tbsp. - optional
- Broccoli – 2 cups **
- Shredded cheddar cheese - .75 cups
- Pepper and salt – to your liking
- Diced green onions - 2

Use either fresh and steamed or defrosted and frozen broccoli.

Preparation Method:

1. Warm up the oven to 350°F. Prepare 6 muffin tins with paper liners or cooking spray.
2. Whisk all of the eggs, salt, pepper, and mustard. Blend in the green onions, broccoli, and cheese.
3. Divide up the batter and bake for 12-14 minutes.
4. Serve when they are puffy and thoroughly cooked.

Cinnamon-Apple French Toast

Freestyle Points: 4

Yields: 4 Servings

Ingredients:

- Liquid egg whites – 1.33 cups
- 1% milk – 1 cup
- Eggs – 4
- Cinnamon – 2 tsp.
- Apples – 2
- Slices of low-calorie bread – 8
- Also Needed: 9 x 13 casserole dish

Preparation Method:

1. Peel and dice the apples. Grease the baking dish with cooking spray. Prepare the oven temperature to 350°F.
2. Using a microwavable dish to combine and cook the cinnamon and apples for three minutes.
3. Line the baking dish with bread slices and a layer of cooked apples.
4. Whisk the egg whites and milk. Pour over the bread. Bake 45 minutes. Serve and enjoy with your favorite toppings.

Country Cottage Pancakes

Freestyle Points: 3

Yields: 4 Servings

Ingredients:

- Low-fat cottage cheese – 1 cup
- Medium eggs – 8
- Coconut flour – 4 tbsp.
- Bicarb of soda - .5 tsp.
- Almond flour – 4 tbsp.
- Grated zest of lemon – 1 tsp.
- Kosher salt – A pinch
- Vanilla essence - .5 tsp.
- Sweetened almond milk – 4 tbsp.

Preparation Method:

1. In a blender; combine all of the fixings – excluding the almond milk for now. Blitz until smooth.
2. Lightly spritz a skillet with cooking oil spray. Warm it up using medium-high temperature setting.
3. Prepare in four batches – one at a time. Flip only once, when the pancakes start bubbling. Continue cooking and serve immediately.

Egg & Sausage Muffins

Freestyle Points: 1

Yields: 20 Servings

Ingredients:

- Lean turkey breakfast sausage – 1 lb.
- Liquid egg whites – 3 cups
- Minced cloves of garlic - 2
- Green chilis – 4 oz. – 1 can - mild or hot
- Small chopped onion - 1
- Hash browns – 3 cups
- Black pepper – to your liking
- Sea salt – 1.5 tsp.

Preparation Method:

1. Warm up the oven to 375°F. Prepare 20 muffin tins with some cooking spray.
2. Cook the sausage on the stovetop using the med-high heat setting. As it breaks apart, stir in the onions, garlic, and chilies. Remove when the onions have softened.
3. Prepare the same skillet with a spritz of cooking spray. Toss in the hash browns, salt, and pepper the way you like it. Simmer 3-4 minutes. Fold in the eggs and combine well.
4. Dump the prepared batter into the tins. Bake 15-18 minutes. Check the centers for doneness using the toothpick test.

Egg & Veggie Scramble

Freestyle Points: 1

Yields: 6 Servings

Ingredients:

- Extra-virgin olive oil – 1.5 tbsp.
- Diced tomato - 1
- Large eggs - 6
- Baby spinach – 3 cups
- Minced garlic clove - 1
- Red or purple diced onion - .5 of 1
- Black pepper and Kosher salt – 1 tsp. of each
- 2% sharp cheddar cheese - .5 cup

Preparation Method:

1. Whisk the eggs, pepper, and salt.
2. Warm up the olive oil in a skillet. Toss in the spinach, tomato, onions, and garlic. Simmer until done or about 5-7 minutes.
3. Pour in the eggs and simmer 3-4 minutes – stirring occasionally. When set, remove from the burner and add the cheese on top. Serve and enjoy.

Hard-Boiled Eggs in the Instant Pot

Freestyle Points: -0-

Yields: Varies

Ingredients:

- Water – 1 cup
- Eggs - your choice in a single layer

Preparation Method:

1. Measure out the water and add to the pot. Gently add the eggs to the rack basket. Close the lid and set the timer for 3-5 minutes (high-pressure).
2. Natural release the pressure for 5 minutes and quick release the remainder of the built-up steam pressure.
3. Arrange the eggs in a cold-water dish to cool. A few ice cubes will speed the process. Wait 5-10 minutes before peeling.

Muffin Tin Eggs

Freestyle Points: 1

Yields: 6 Servings

Ingredients

- Eggs – 1 dozen
- Fat-free ground turkey breast - .5 lb.
- Diced green bell pepper – 1
- Steak seasoning – ex. Montreal Blend – 1 tsp.
- Red pepper flakes - .25 tsp.
- Black pepper and salt - .5 tsp. each
- Sage - .5 tsp.
- Marjoram - .25 tsp.
- Also Needed: -12-cup muffin tin

Preparation Method:

1. Set the oven temperature to 350°F. Prepare the muffin tin with cooking spray.
2. Spray the skillet and add the turkey, pepper flakes, black pepper, marjoram, salt, and sage. Cook for 7-10 minutes. Stir often to prevent sticking.
3. In a large mixing container, combine the steak seasoning and eggs - mixing well (2-3 min.) until fluffy. Blend in the diced pepper.
4. Once the turkey mixture is done, spoon into the tins and add the egg mixture. Fill about 3/4 full and bake for 30 minutes in the hot oven.

Tropical Breakfast Pie

Freestyle Points: 5

Yields: 4 Servings

Ingredients:

- Refrigerated biscuit dough – 7.5 oz.

- Unsweetened shredded coconut – 2 tbsp.

- Granulated sugar - .5 tsp.

- Fresh pineapple – 1 cup

- Also Needed: 8-inch-square casserole dish

Preparation Method:

1. Warm up the oven in advance to 350°F.

2. Lightly coat the casserole dish with a splash of cooking spray. Break apart the dough into 10 portions and slice into quarters.

3. Load a Ziploc-type bag with the sugar and coconut. Shake well and add the dough bits. Shake gently, but well to coat.

4. Place the biscuits into the dish and garnish with the diced pineapple.

5. Place in the preheated oven. Bake for 25 minutes.

Zucchini Noodles & Poached Eggs – Instant Pot

Freestyle Points: 4

Yields: 3 Servings

Ingredients for the Noodles:

- Olive oil – 1 tsp.
- Large spiralized zucchinis – 2
- Chopped cauliflower – 1 cup
- Garlic cloves – 2
- Small chopped onion – 1
- Large eggs – 2

Ingredients for the Seasoning:

- Ground smoked paprika - .5 tsp.
- Salt – 1 tsp.
- Black pepper - .5 tsp.
- Finely chopped chives – 1 tsp.
- Also Needed: Spiralizer

Preparation Method:

1. Rinse the zucchinis and discard the tips. Spiralize and set aside.
2. Plug in the Instant Pot. Give it a spritz of the olive oil in the stainless-steel insert. Add in the noodles and water and cook for 5 minutes. Set aside and cover.
3. Stir in the chopped cauliflower with a sprinkle of salt. Pour enough water to cover, and secure the top. Set the timer for 5 minutes using

the high-pressure setting.

4. Quick release the pressure and add to the food processor with the salt, pepper, paprika, onion, and garlic. Blend until smooth.

5. Return the rest of the fixings into the Instant Pot and stir. Add the eggs on top and saute for around 3 minutes or until the eggs are cooked to your preference. Serve with a sprinkle of chives.

Chapter 3: Lunch favorites

Whether you want some quick chicken, a bowl of soup or a salad; you'll find it here!

CHICKEN

Asian Turkey Stir-Fry

Freestyle Points: 2

Yields: 4 Servings

Ingredients:

- Asian vegetable mix - 16 oz. bag
- Ground turkey - 99% lean - 1 lb.
- Soy sauce – 4 tbsp.
- Minced cloves of garlic – 2
- Minced ginger – 2 tbsp.
- Coconut oil – 1 tbsp.
- Rice vinegar – 2 tbsp.
- Sesame oil – 1 tbsp.

Preparation Method:

1. Warm up the oil using med-high heat. Next, add the turkey, garlic, and ginger.
2. After the turkey is fully cooked; just dump the veggies into the pan. Next, cook it for 4 to 5 minutes or until tender.
3. Pour in the soy sauce and vinegar. Cook for two more minutes. Taste and add seasoning or soy sauce as desired before serving.

Buffalo Chicken Tenders

Freestyle Points: 5

Yields: 6 Servings

Ingredients:

- Chicken breasts – 1 lb.
- Panko breadcrumbs – 1 cup
- Flour - .25 cup
- Eggs – 3
- Red hot sauce - .33 cup
- Brown sugar - .5 cup
- Garlic powder - .5 tsp.
- Water – 3 tbsp.

Preparation Method:

1. Set the oven setting to 425°F.
2. Slice the chicken into strips and pound to 1/2-inch thickness for even cooking and tenderness. Toss into a zipper-type baggie along with the flour. Shake well.
3. Add the breadcrumbs in one dish and the eggs in another.
4. Dredge the chicken in the eggs, then the breadcrumbs. Arrange on a baking sheet and spray with a misting of cooking oil. Bake 20 minutes.
5. Prepare the sauce with the rest of the fixings in a small saucepan.
6. Enjoy the tenders with the sauce and your favorite side of veggies.

SALADS

Caesar Salad – Instant Pot

Freestyle Points: 5

Yields: 5 Servings

Ingredients:

- Chicken breasts – 1 lb.
- Iceberg lettuce – 1 cup
- Pepper & Salt – to taste

Ingredients for the Dressing:

- Crushed garlic cloves - 2
- Greek yogurt - .25 cup
- Low-fat mayonnaise – 2 tsp.
- White wine vinegar – 1 tbsp.
- Freshly grated Italian Grana Padano cheese – 2 oz.

Preparation Method:

1. Combine the dressing fixings and set to the side.
2. Prepare the Instant Pot insert and spritz with some cooking oil. Warm it up using the saute function. Add the chicken with the pepper and salt. Saute three to four minutes per side. Take it out of the pot and set those aside also.
3. Roughly chop the lettuce and toss in the chicken with a sprinkle of the dressing.
4. Serve immediately and enjoy.

Ham Salad

Freestyle Points: 2

Yields: 4 Servings

Ingredients:

- Cooked – chopped ham – 1 cup
- Mango chutney – 1 tbsp.
- Onion powder – 2 tsp.
- Light mayonnaise – 2 tbsp.
- Dried mustard – 2 tsp.
- Non-fat plain Greek yogurt – 2 tbsp.

Preparation Method:

1. Pulse the fixings (omit the ham or not) in a processor until smooth.
2. Place the container in the refrigerator for about 30 minutes.
3. Add a dish of cucumber slices for a -0- points.

Pear & Blue Cheese Salad

Freestyle Points: 3

Servings: 4

Ingredients:

- White wine vinegar – 2 tbsp.
- Pear nectar - .25 cup
- Walnut oil – 2 tbsp.
- Ground black pepper - .125 tsp.
- Ground ginger - .125 tsp.
- Medium green pears – sliced - 3
- Torn mesclun greens – 10 cups
- Dijon mustard – 1 tsp.
- Honey – 1 tsp.
- Broken walnuts - .5 cup
- Crumbled blue cheese - .5 cup

Preparation Method:

1. Whisk the walnut oil, nectar, vinegar, honey, pepper, ginger, and mustard until well mixed. Set to the side for now.
2. Combine the rest of the ingredients and add the dressing. Toss well to coat. Chill in the fridge before time to eat.

Tuna Salad with Cranberries – Onion & Celery

Freestyle Points: 3

Yields: 5 Servings

Ingredients for the Seasoning – to taste:

- Red pepper flakes
- Freshly cracked black pepper
- Sea salt

Ingredients for the Tuna Salad:

- White tuna in spring water – 16 oz. can
- Low-fat mayonnaise – 3 tbsp.
- Light sour cream – 3 tbsp.
- Celery - .5 cup
- Red onion - .25 cup
- Dried cranberries - .25 cup
- Lemon juice – 1 tbsp.
- Cored apple - 1

Preparation Method:

1. Drain the tuna, mince the onion, and chop the celery. Core and thinly slice the apples.
2. Squeeze a fresh lemon for fresh juice. Combine the seasonings. Also, combine the salad fixings.
3. When ready to serve, garnish as desired and enjoy.

SOUPS

Beef Chili – Slow-Cooker

Freestyle Points: 4

Yields: 12 Servings

Ingredients:

- Lean ground beef – 1 lb.
- Diced bell peppers - 2
- Minced cloves of garlic
- Cumin – 2 tsp.
- Diced tomatoes – 1 can – 28 oz.
- Green chilis – canned .25 cup
- Kidney beans – 15 oz.
- Onion – 1 chopped
- Chili powder – 2 tbsp.
- Tomato paste – 2 tbsp.
- Salt – to taste

Preparation Method:

1. Warm up a skillet using the med-high temperature setting. Stir in the garlic and beef until browned (10 min. or so). Stir in the peppers and continue cooking 5 more minutes. Sprinkle with the cumin and chili powder.

2. Scoop the meat into the slow cooker with the remainder of the fixings. Stir and close the top. Prepare for eight to ten hours using the low-temperature setting.

3. When done, just taste test and adjust the seasonings to your liking.

Butternut Squash Soup

Freestyle Points: 1

Yields: 8 Servings

Ingredients:

- Raw cubed squash – 12 oz.

- Fat-free vegetable stock – 4 cups

- Green apple - .5 of 1

- Onion - .5 of 1

- Ground ginger – 1 pinch

- Black pepper & Salt – to taste

- Ground nutmeg – 1 pinch

Preparation Method:

1. Warm up a large stockpot and add the apple, onion, squash, and stock. Stir and cover until it boils. Then, reduce the temperature and remove the lid.

2. Continue cooking slowly for 10 minutes and puree with a blender. Give it a shake of salt, pepper, nutmeg, and ginger.

3. Serve and enjoy.

Chicken-Parmesan Soup

Freestyle Points: 3

Yields: 8 Servings

Ingredients:

- Olive oil – 1 tbsp.
- Minced cloves of garlic - 3
- Diced onion - 1
- Crushed tomatoes – 15 oz.
- Chicken stock – 6 cups
- Chicken breasts- no bones or skin – 12 oz.
- Part-skim mozzarella cheese – 1.5 cups
- Grated parmesan – 2 tbsp.
- Salt – 1 tsp.
- Red pepper flakes - .5 tsp.
- Dried parsley – 1 tsp.
- Black pepper - .5 tsp.

Preparation Method:

1. Prepare the stockpot using the med-high setting and add the oil. When warm, toss in the onions. Simmer 6 minutes. Toss in the garlic and continue cooking one additional minute.
2. Stir in the stock and tomatoes. Once it boils; just lower the heat setting. Remove the skin and bones from the chicken and add to the pot with the rest of the ingredients.
3. Simmer until the cheese is melted and serve.

Fish & Shrimp Stew

Freestyle Points: 2

Yields: 6 Servings

Ingredients:

- Minced garlic cloves - 2
- Crushed tomatoes – 28 oz. can
- Diced onion - 1
- Olive oil – 1 tbsp.
- Tomato paste – 3 tbsp.
- Parsley - .66 cup
- Fish stock – 14 oz.
- Clam juice – 8 oz.
- Ghee or butter – 2 tbsp.
- Basil – 5 tsp.
- Oregano - .5 tsp.
- Red pepper flakes - .25 tsp.
- Pepper and salt – to taste
- Raw shrimp – 1 lb.
- Cod – 2-inch pieces – 1.5 lb.

Preparation Method:

1. Use the medium heat setting to heat up the oil in a skillet. Toss in the onion and cook for five to seven minutes. Stir in the pepper flakes and garlic. Cook for another one to two minutes. Pour in the tomato paste and simmer one additional minute.

2. Stir in the tomatoes, clam juice, and fish stock. Simmer and add the basil, oregano, and butter. Simmer for 10-15 minutes.

3. Taste test and add the cod. Simmer for another 5 minutes and fold in the shrimp.

4. Continue cooking for 4-5 minutes until the shrimp is opaque.

5. Serve and enjoy.

Lentil Soup – Instant Pot

Freestyle Points: 1

Yield: 6 servings

Ingredients:

- Yellow onion - 1
- Carrots - 2
- Celery stalks - 2
- Diced tomatoes with juice – 1 can 15 oz.
- Garlic cloves - 2
- Curry powder – 1 tsp.
- Optional: Cayenne pepper - 1 pinch
- Ground cumin – 1 tsp.
- Dry green or brown lentils – 1 cup
- Water – 3 cups
- Freshly cracked black pepper – to taste
- Salt – 1 tsp. or more
- Fresh spinach - roughly chopped – 1 cup
- For Serving: Lemon slices

Preparation Method:

1. Plug in the Instant Pot to warm up for 10-15 minutes.
2. Peel and chop the onions, celery, and carrots. Mince the cloves of garlic and roughly chop the spinach.
3. Combine in the Instant Pot; the water, lentils, cayenne, curry, cumin, garlic, tomatoes, celery, onions, carrots, and a dash of black pepper. Stir

well. (Omit the salt)

4. Close the top and lock it down. Set the timer for 10 minutes using the high-pressure setting. When it's done; just natural release the pressure for about 10 minutes and open the lid.

5. Stir and make sure the soup is well done. Add 1 teaspoon of salt with the spinach.

6. Serve warm after the spinach wilts. Garnish with a lemon wedge. Serve any time for up to a week when stored in the fridge in an air-tight container.

Vegetable Soup

Freestyle Points: -0-

Yields: 6 Servings

Ingredients:

- Minced cloves of garlic - 3
- Chopped onion - 1
- Chicken stock - fat-free – 3 cups
- Frozen spinach – 10 oz.
- Diced zucchini - .5 cup
- Green beans - .5 cup
- Chopped carrots - .5 cup
- Tomato paste – 1 tbsp.
- Salt & Black pepper – to your liking
- Italian seasoning – 1 tsp.

Preparation Method:

1. Lightly spray a saucepan with some cooking oil spray. Warm it up using the medium heat setting and toss in the onion and garlic.
2. Cook about five minutes and stir in the tomato paste, stock, carrots, and green beans. Prepare for about 6 minutes.
3. Fold in the zucchini and simmer 5 additional minutes before adding the spinach to cook until heated.
4. Season to your liking and serve.

Chapter 4: Scrumptious dinner choices: Beef – Fish & Seafood

Dinnertime is a special time of the day where your family can sit down and enjoy the conversations of daily events. From beef to fish and seafood, you will find a tempting dish to fit any occasion.

BEEF CHOICES

Beef & Broccoli Stir-Fry

Freestyle Points: 3

Yields: 4 Servings

Ingredients:

- Lean sirloin beef - .75 lb.
- Table salt - .25 tsp.
- Cornstarch – divided – 2.5 tbsp.
- Canola oil – 2 tsp.
- Broccoli florets - 12 oz. bag – 5 cups
- Chicken broth – reduced-sodium – divided – 1 cup
- Minced garlic – 2 tbsp.
- Soy sauce - .25 cup
- Water - .25 cup
- Red pepper flakes - .25 tsp.
- Minced ginger root – 1 tbsp.

Preparation Method:

1. Combine two tablespoons of the cornstarch with the salt and add the beef to coat.

2. Warm up the oil in a wok or deep skillet using the med-hi heat setting.

3. Add the beef and cook for four minutes. Transfer to a bowl.

4. In the same pan, pour one-half cup of the broth and loosen the bits on the bottom. Fold in the broccoli and add one tbsp. of water - if needed. Cook for three minutes with the lid on.

5. Add the garlic, ginger, and pepper flakes. Simmer one more minute.

6. In a mixing cup, combine the rest of the broth, soy sauce, and remainder of the cornstarch. Pour into the pan and lower the temperature setting to med-low. Simmer one more minute and return the juices and beef into the pan. Toss to coat well and serve.

Beef & Mushrooms – Slow Cooker

Freestyle Points: 5

Yields: 6 Servings

Ingredients:

- Lean stewing beef meat – 2 lb.
- Olive oil – 2 tsp.
- Fresh mushrooms – 10 oz.
- Cream of mushroom soup – low-sodium/fat-free – 10.75 oz can
- Soup mix – dry onion – 1 envelope
- Dry red wine - .5 cup
- Suggested Cooker Size: 4-Quarts

Preparation Method:

1. Use the medium heat setting to warm up a skillet.
2. Do the Prep: Cube the stewing beef and slice the mushrooms.
3. Sprinkle the beef with the pepper and salt to your liking. Arrange it in the pan. Layer evenly and brown. Add to the cooker.
4. Brown the mushrooms and toss them into the pot.
5. Stir in the wine and scrape up the browned crunchies. Pour in the soup and soup mix. Mix well and cover.
6. Simmer on low for six to eight hours. Serve when ready.

Jalapeno Popper Burgers

Freestyle Points: 6

Yields: 4 Servings

Ingredients:

- 1 1/3 lb. ground beef – 1.33 lb.
- Finely chopped jalapeno - 1
- Cream cheese - reduced-fat – 2 tbsp.
- Mustard – 2 tsp.
- Worcestershire sauce – 2 tsp.
- Shredded cheddar cheese - .5 cup
- Kosher salt – divided – 5 tsp.

Preparation Method:

1. Combine all of the burger fixings. Divide into six patties and wait about 10 minutes before cooking for the flavors to mix.
2. Grill to your liking (4-6 min. per side suggested). If you prefer, use a skillet and cook for 5-6 minutes for each side.
3. Note: You can also use ground turkey.

Spicy Beef & Zucchini Skillet

Freestyle Points: 6

Yields: 4 Servings

Ingredients:

- Ground beef - lean – 1 lb.
- Olive oil – 1 tsp.
- Minced garlic cloves - 3
- Chopped onion - 1
- Green chilis - 1 can – 4 oz.
- Diced tomatoes - 14 oz. – 2 cans of each
- Drained black beans – 2 cans 14 oz. each
- Lime – juice of 1
- Chili powder – 1 tbsp.
- Chopped zucchinis - 2
- Ground black pepper & Salt – to taste

Preparation Method:

1. Use the med-high setting on the stovetop to heat up the oil.
2. Once it's hot, toss in the onions and garlic. Saute two minutes and add the beef. Once it is browning, stir in the chilis, beans, tomatoes, lime juice, chili powder, pepper, and salt.
3. Continue cooking for 10 minutes. Take off the top and add the chopped zucchini. Cook 10 more minutes and serve.

FISH & SEAFOOD

Apple Trout

Freestyle Points: 3

Yields: 4 Servings

Ingredients:

- Soy sauce – 1 tsp.
- Freshly squeezed lemon juice – 1 tsp.
- Rice vinegar – 1 tsp.
- Granny Smith apple – 1 Medium
- Trout fillets – 7 oz.

Ingredients for the Seasoning Ingredients:

- Black pepper - .5 tsp
- Sea salt - .5 tsp
- Fresh parsley – 1 tbsp.
- Ground dried rosemary - .25 tsp.

Preparation Method:

1. Cut the apple and fillets into bite-sized pieces and squeeze the lemon juice.
2. Whisk the vinegar, lemon juice, soy sauce, rosemary, salt, pepper, and parsley in a mixing dish. Brush the trout.
3. Lightly grease the Instant Pot and add the oil. Using the saute function, add the apple and fish. Prepare 2 minutes. Add enough water to cover and secure the lid.
4. Set the timer for 2 minutes using the high-pressure setting. When the

time is completed, open the lid and vent the steam.

5. Serve with your favorite 'zero' veggie.

Cajun Salmon

Freestyle Points: 1

Yields: 4 Servings

Ingredients:

- Olive oil – 1 tbsp.
- Salmon – 1.33 lb.
- Dried thyme - .25 tsp.
- Salt and Pepper - .5 tsp. each
- Paprika – 2 tsp.
- Onion powder - .5 tsp.
- Cayenne - .125 tsp.
- Garlic powder - .5 tsp.

Preparation Method:

1. Combine the spices to make the seasoning.
2. Brush the salmon with oil and a drizzle of the seasoning.
3. On the Grill: Arrange the salmon, so that the skin is facing downwards. Cook three to four minutes. Turn the salmon over and continue cooking for an additional 1-3 minutes. Choose a delicious side dish and serve.

Chapter 5: Scrumptious dinner choices: Pork & poultry

PORK

Cuban Pork – Instant Pot

Freestyle Points: 5

Yields: 10 Servings

Ingredients:

- Garlic cloves – 6
- Pork shoulder blade roast – boneless – 3 lb.
- Bay leaf – 1
- Kosher salt – 1 tbsp.
- Lime juice - .66 cup
- Grapefruit juice- .66 cup
- Fresh oregano – 5 tbsp.
- Cumin – 5 tbsp.

Ingredients for Serving:

- Salsa
- Lime wedges
- Chopped cilantro
- Hot sauce
- Tortillas

Preparation Method:

1. Chop the meat into four pieces and place in a mixing container.

2. Use a mini food processor and combine both of the juices, garlic, salt, cumin, and oregano. Blend until smooth.

3. Pour the mixture over the shoulder pieces and let it marinate one hour on the countertop. You can also marinate overnight in the refrigerator.

4. When ready to prepare; add the meat to the cooker along with the bay leaf.

5. Cook using the high-pressure setting for 80 minutes. Natural release the pressure.

6. Shred the meat and remove the juices from the Instant Pot/pressure cooker.

7. Pour one cup of the juices and add the meat back into the pot. Season to taste. Keep it warm until serving time.

Pork Chops with Creamy Sauce

Freestyle Points: 5

Yields: 4 Servings

Ingredients:

- Pork loin chops - center-cut – 4 - Approximately 4 oz. ea.
- Non-fat Half-and-Half - .33 cup
- Fat-free chicken stock - .33 cup
- Black pepper - .5 tsp.
- Onion powder - .5 tsp.
- Salt - .5 tsp.
- Dijon mustard – 1.5 tbsp.
- Dried thyme – 1 pinch

Preparation Method:

1. Shake the salt, pepper, and onion powder over the chops.
2. Using the med-high heat setting on the stovetop, prepare a large skillet with cooking spray.
3. Once the pan is hot, add the chops and fry for 3-4 minutes per side. The internal temperature should reach a minimum temperature on a meat thermometer of 145°F.
4. At this point; just place the prepared chops in a closed container and keep them warm.
5. Pour the chicken stock into the skillet and deglaze the browned bits. Stir in the mustard and Half-and-Half.
6. Lower the temperature setting to medium and continue cooking for 7 minutes. When the sauce has thickened, add the thyme.
7. Serve with the sauce and your favorite side dish.

Raspberry Pork Chops in the Crock Pot

Freestyle Points: 8

Yields: 4 servings

Ingredients:

- Boneless pork chops – 4 – 4 oz. each
- Seasonings: Pepper – salt – meat seasoning; ex. Montreal Steak
- Chicken broth - .25 cup
- Raspberry jam - .75 cup
- Balsamic vinegar – 3 tbsp.
- Chopped chipotle pepper in adobo sauce – 1 tsp.
- Suggested Cooker Size: 4-quarts

Preparation Method:

1. Lightly grease the slow cooker. Whisk the finely chopped chipotle, vinegar, broth, and jam.
2. Season the pork chops to your liking and add two of them to the cooker. Add the sauce and the last two chops with the rest of the sauce.
3. Secure the top and cook 4-6 hours on the low setting.
4. Enjoy with a salad or dish of brown rice.

POULTRY

Cheesy Southwestern Chicken – Slow Cooker

Freestyle Points: 1

Yields: 6 Servings

Ingredients:

- Chunky salsa – 16 oz. – 1 jar - divided
- Chicken breast halves - 6
- Corn – 15.5 oz. ea. – 2 cans
- Black beans - 15 oz. – 1 can
- Low-fat shredded Mexican cheese blend – 1 cup
- Optional: Southwest seasoning blend
- Suggested: 5-6-quart slow cooker

Preparation Method:

1. Rinse and drain the corn and black beans. Add to the slow cooker with about half of the salsa.
2. Remove the bones and skin from the chicken. Shake with the salt and pepper or seasoning blend if using.
3. Add the chicken to the pot and the rest of the salsa. Secure the lid and cook on the low-temperature setting until tender (4-6 hrs.).
4. Sprinkle with the cheese. Cover again to melt the cheese (5 min.).

Italian – Balsamic Chicken

Freestyle Points: 1

Yields: 4 Servings

Ingredients:

- Breasts of chicken – 1.33 lb.
- Salt and pepper – 1 tsp. each
- Italian seasoning – 2 tsp.
- Balsamic vinegar – 2.5 tbsp.
- Olive oil – 2 tsp.
- Minced garlic cloves - 3
- Sliced mushrooms - 8 oz.
- Chicken stock - .5 cup

Preparation Method:

1. Combine the salt, pepper, and Italian seasoning. Sprinkle the chicken.
2. Warm up a skillet with the oil using the med-high heat setting. When ready, add the seasoned chicken. Simmer slowly for two to three minutes on each side. Put it to the side for now.
3. Toss the garlic and mushrooms into the pan and saute three to four minutes. Stir in the vinegar and chicken stock. Stir well and deglaze the pan. Toss the chicken in the sauce and simmer about 10 to 15 minutes until done.
4. Note: Be sure to use high-quality balsamic vinegar for the best results.

Oven-Baked Chicken Kebabs – Slow Cooker

Freestyle Points: 2

Yields: 4 Servings

Ingredients:

- Olive oil – 2 tbsp.
- Fresh parsley - .25 cup
- Taco seasoning – 1 tsp.
- Salt – 1 tsp.
- Minced cloves of garlic - 3
- Boneless chicken breasts – 1.33 lb.
- Yellow - red or mixed bell peppers - 2
- Cherry tomatoes – a small handful
- Onion – 1 small
- Juiced limes - 2

Preparation Method:

1. Cut the onion and peppers into chunks. Juice the lime.
2. Add the taco seasoning, salt, garlic, oil, juice of the lime, and parsley in a blender. Process until it's smooth.
3. Cube the chicken and shake in the bag of prepared marinade. Store in the fridge for about 30 minutes.
4. When ready to prepare, warm up the oven broiler.
5. Arrange the chicken tomatoes, peppers, and onions on skewers.
6. Add the prepared kebabs onto a baking tin.
7. Bake for 5 minutes and flip. Broil for another 5 minutes.
8. Serve when the chicken reaches an internal temperature of 165°F.
9. Note: You can add other fixings to the kebabs if you have some extras on hand. (Be sure to check for any additional points.)

Pesto Baked Chicken

Freestyle Points: 3

Yields: 4 Servings

What You Need:

- Butterflied chicken breasts – 1 lb.
- Pesto - .25 cup
- Low-fat grated mozzarella cheese - .5 cup
- Cherry tomatoes- 1 cup
- Sea salt & Freshly cracked black pepper – to your liking

Preparation Method:

1. Cut away all of the bones and skin from the chicken. Slice the tomatoes into halves.
2. Warm up the oven to 400°F. Prepare a baking tin with a sheet of aluminum foil and a spritz of non-stick spray.
3. Coat with the pepper and salt with a spread of the pesto.
4. Place on the baking tin with the tomatoes. Bake 15-17 minutes.
5. Take it out of the oven and drizzle with the cheese. Bake another 5-6 minutes until the cheese is lightly browned.

Chapter 6: Delicious sides

Pair off one of these delicious dishes with your main course.

SIDES

Asparagus Sauteed with Bacon

Freestyle Points: 1

Yields: 4 Servings – .66 cup each

Ingredients:

- Medium sliced shallot - 1
- Asparagus – 1 lb.
- Sea salt - .25 tsp.
- Freshly cracked black pepper - .125 tsp.
- Center-cut bacon – 4 slices
- White wine vinegar – 1.5 tsp.

Preparation Method:

1. Slice the bacon into small pieces. Prepare in a skillet for 5 minutes. Remove and drain on a paper towel. Leave only one teaspoon of grease in the pan and pour the rest in a jar for later or discard.
2. Trim and dice the asparagus into chunks and slice the shallots. Add to the pan and saute about 7 minutes, stirring frequently.
3. Toss the bacon, pepper, and salt over the mixture using the med-high temperature until warm.
4. Transfer to serving dishes and stir in the vinegar.

Brown Sugar Baked Beans – Instant Pot

Freestyle Points: 2

Yield: 8 servings

Ingredients:

- Finely diced yellow onion - 1
- Northern beans -approx. 1.75 cups
- Kidney beans - 1 can – 15.5 oz. - approx. 1.75 cups
- Pinto beans - 1 can or approx. 1.75 cups
- Chili powder - 1 tsp.
- Water - .75 cup
- Ketchup - .5 cup
- Dark brown sugar – not packed - .33 cup
- Yellow mustard – 1 tbsp.

Preparation Method:

1. Rinse and drain the beans. Combine all of the fixings in the Instant Pot. Secure the lid and lock. Use the manual setting on high-pressure for 8 minutes.
2. Natural release the pressure when the time has elapsed (10-15 minutes) or quick release if you are in a hurry. Stir before serving.

Caesar Green Beans

Freestyle Points: 2

Yields: 4 Servings

Ingredients for the Beans:

- Water – 2 cups
- Green beans – 1 lb.
- Low-cal Caesar dressing – 1.5 tbsp.
- Shredded parmesan cheese – 1 tbsp.

Ingredients for the Crumb Topping:

- Powdered garlic – 1 tsp.
- Low-cal butter – 1 tsp.
- Whole grain toast – 1 slice

Preparation Method:

1. Trim the green beans and shred the cheese.
2. Toss the greens into a pot of boiling water. Simmer until tender (5 min.). Add to a colander to remove the liquids.
3. Butter the toast and sprinkle with the garlic. Microwave 10 minutes and add to a food processor. Blitz until crumbly.
4. Serve the beans with a sprinkle of the crumbs and a serving of dressing. Sprinkle with the parmesan and serve.

Creamy Broccoli – Instant Pot

Freestyle Points – 4

Yields: 4 Servings

Ingredients:

- Vegetable stock – 2 cups
- Chopped broccoli – 1 lb.
- Halved brussels sprouts – 1 cup
- Sliced red onion – 1 medium-sized
- Minced cloves of garlic – 2
- Salt - .5 tsp.

Ingredients for the Sauce:

- Soy sauce – 1 tbsp.
- Freshly squeezed lime juice – 1 tsp.
- Heavy cream – 2 tbsp.
- Olive oil – 1 tbsp.
- Ground black pepper & salt - .5 tsp. each
- Freshly ground ginger - .25 tsp.
- Also Needed: Food Processor

Preparation Method:

1. Add the brussels sprouts and broccoli to the stainless-steel insert of the Instant Pot. Pour in the vegetable stock and salt.
2. Close the lid and choose the high-pressure setting for five minutes.

3. When the timer buzzes, quick release the pressure and remove the veggies with a slotted spoon.

4. Prep the food processor by adding the garlic, onions, and each of the sauce fixings. Pulse until the mixture is creamy.

5. Select the saute function and pour the prepared sauce into the insert. Let it simmer for five minutes. Stir occasionally.

6. Serve over the veggies and enjoy!

Mashed Sweet Potatoes

Freestyle Points: 2

Servings: 4

Ingredients:

- Large sweet potatoes - 2
- Salt & Black pepper - .5 tsp of each
- Garlic powder – 1 tsp.
- Plain fat-free Greek yogurt - .5 cup

Preparation Method:

1. Wash, peel, and cube the potatoes. Prepare a pot of boiling water (enough to cover the potatoes). Add the potatoes. Boil using the med-high stovetop setting for 8-10 minutes.

2. Dump the potatoes into a colander to drain and add to a large mixing container. Combine with the seasonings and yogurt.

3. Use a hand mixer or mix by hand to mash the fixings until smooth.

Pinto Beans - Crockpot

Freestyle Points: -0-

Yields: 8 Servings

Ingredients:

- Onion - 1
- Dry pinto beans – 1 lb.
- Bay leaves - 2
- Garlic cloves - 4
- Poblano peppers - 2
- Salt – 1 tsp.
- Cumin - .5 tbsp.
- Water or broth – to cover the beans – 6 cups

Preparation Method:

1. Dice the garlic, peppers, and onion. Rinse the beans thoroughly and add to the crockpot.
2. Toss in the rest of the fixings and cover with broth or water. It should be at least one inch over the beans.
3. Prepare for 8-10 hours using the low setting. Times vary with each cooker. When done, the beans will be soft and tasty.

Rainbow Potato Salad

Freestyle Points: 4

Yields: 6 Servings

Ingredients for the Potatoes:

- Yellow potatoes – 1 lb.
- Purple potatoes- .5 lb.
- Red potatoes- .5 lb.

Ingredients for the Dressing:

- Fresh dill - .5 cup
- Scallions - .5 cup
- Celery – 1 stalk
- Low-calorie ranch dressing - .5 cup
- Salt and pepper – to taste

Preparation Method:

1. Cube the potatoes. Finely chop the scallions and celery. Roughly chop the dill.
2. Add all of the potatoes to a pan full of water. Boil and cover. Continue to cook until softened (10-12 min.).
3. Drain the water out of the potatoes and let cool.
4. Combine the dressing fixings in a mixing container. When cool, add the potatoes and stir until incorporated.
5. Chill in the fridge or serve warm.

Roasted Carrots

Freestyle Points: 2

Yields: 4 Servings

Ingredients:

- Baby carrots - 1 bag – 16 oz.
- Dried parsley - .25 tsp.
- Salt - .25 tsp.
- Black pepper – 1 pinch
- Ginger - .25 tsp.
- Cinnamon – 1 pinch
- Olive oil – 1.5 tbsp.
- Also Needed: 9 x 13 casserole dish

Preparation Method:

1. Warm up the oven to 450°F.
2. Prepare the baking dish with the oil and carrots. Sprinkle with the fixings. Bake for 20-25 minutes until tender.
3. Serve with your favorite main dish.

In the next segment, you will discover how easy it is to prepare a days-worth of meals and stay within your desired goals. Once you know how many points you can add to your menu plan (your personal total of allowed points), feel free to add up to those limits and enjoy the freedom provided by your new way of life. Each day has the total provided for points allowed for each recipe item and a daily total.

Chapter 7: 21-day meal plan

DAY 1:

- Breakfast: Baked Omelet – 2
- Lunch: Fish & Shrimp Stew – 2
- Dinner: Beef & Broccoli Stir-Fry – 3

Totals - Day 1: 7

DAY 2:

- Breakfast: Banana Roll-Ups – 2
- Lunch: Buffalo Chicken Tenders – 5
- Lunch Side: Asparagus Sauteed with Bacon – 1
- Dinner: Apple Trout – 3
- Dinner: Side: Brown Sugar Baked Beans – Instant Pot - 2

Totals – Day 2: 13

DAY 3:

- Breakfast: Broccoli Cheddar Egg Muffins - 2
- Lunch: Caesar Salad – Instant Pot – 5
- Dinner: Cheesy Southwestern Chicken – Slow Cooker -1
- Dinner Side: Rainbow Potato Salad – 4

Totals - Day 3: 12

DAY 4:

- Breakfast: Cinnamon-Apple French Toast – 4
- Lunch: Asian Turkey Stir-Fry - 2
- Dinner: Cuban Pork – Instant Pot – 5
- Dinner Side: Pinto Beans – Crockpot - 0-

Totals - Day 4: 11

DAY 5:

- Breakfast: Country Cottage Pancakes – 3
- Lunch: Ham Salad – 2
- Lunch Side: Caesar Green Beans – 2
- Dinner: Beef & Mushrooms – Slow Cooker – 5
- Dinner Side: Roasted Carrots - 2

Totals - Day 5: 14

DAY 6:

- Breakfast: Egg & Sausage Muffins – 1
- Lunch: Pear & Blue Cheese Salad - 3
- Dinner: Cajun Salmon – 1
- Dinner Side: Fully-Loaded Macaroni & Cheese with Veggies – 6

Totals - Day 6: 11

DAY 7:

- Breakfast: Egg & Veggie Scramble - 1
- Lunch: Butternut Squash Soup – 1
- Dinner: Jalapeno Popper Burgers – 6

Totals - Day 7: 8

DAY 8:

- Breakfast: Hard-Boiled Eggs in the Instant Pot -0-
- Lunch: Beef Chili – Slow-Cooker - 4
- Dinner: Italian – Balsamic Chicken – 1
- Dinner Side: Leftover - Dinner Side: Fully-Loaded Macaroni & Cheese with Veggies – 6

Totals - Day 8: 11

DAY 9:

- Breakfast: Tropical Breakfast Pie – 5
- Lunch: Asian Turkey Stir-Fry - 2
- Dinner: Italian – Balsamic Chicken – 1
- Dinner Side: Mashed Sweet Potatoes - 2

Totals - Day 9: 10

DAY 10:

- Breakfast: Muffin Tin Eggs – 1
- Lunch: Chicken-Parmesan Soup – 3
- Dinner: Spicy Beef & Zucchini Skillet - 6

Totals - Day 10: 10

DAY 11:

- Breakfast: Zucchini Noodles & Poached Eggs - 4
- Lunch: Tuna Salad with Cranberries – Onion & Celery - 3
- Dinner: Pork Chops with Creamy Sauce – 5
- Dinner Side: Roasted Carrots - 2

Totals – Day 11: 14

DAY 12:

- Breakfast: Baked Omelet – 2
- Lunch: Lentil Soup – Instant Pot – 1
- Dinner: Oven-Baked Chicken Kebabs – Slow Cooker – 2
- Dinner Side: Asparagus Sauteed with Bacon - 1

Totals - Day 12: 6

DAY 13:

- Breakfast: Egg & Sausage Muffins – 1
- Lunch: Fish & Shrimp Stew - 2
- Dinner: Pork Chops with Creamy Sauce – 5
- Dinner Side: Mashed Sweet Potatoes - 2

Totals - Day 13: 10

DAY 14:

- Breakfast: Broccoli Cheddar Egg Muffins - 2
- Lunch: Ham Salad - 2
- Dinner: Pesto Baked Chicken – 3
- Dinner Side: Creamy Broccoli – Instant Pot - 4

Totals - Day 14: 11

DAY 15:

- Breakfast: Banana Roll-Ups – 2
- Lunch: Vegetable Soup -0-
- Dinner: Raspberry Pork Chops in the Crock Pot – 8
- Dinner Side: Caesar Green Beans - 2

Totals - Day 15: 12

DAY 16:

- Breakfast: Cinnamon-Apple French Toast – 4
- Lunch: Butternut Squash Soup – 1
- Dinner: Apple Trout – 3
- Dinner Side: Brown Sugar Baked Beans – Instant Pot - 2

Totals - Day 16: 10

DAY 17:

- Breakfast: Muffin Tin Eggs – 1
- Lunch: Tuna Salad with Cranberries – Onion & Celery - 3
- Dinner: Beef & Broccoli Stir-Fry – 3

Totals - Day 17: 7

DAY 18:

- Breakfast: Egg & Veggie Scramble - 1
- Lunch: Buffalo Chicken Tenders - 5
- Dinner: Cuban Pork – Instant Pot – 5

Totals - Day 18: 11

DAY 19:

- Breakfast: Breakfast: Hard-Boiled Eggs in the Instant Pot –0-
- Lunch: Pear & Blue Cheese Salad - 3
- Dinner: Spicy Beef & Zucchini Skillet - 6

Totals - Day 19: 9

DAY 20:

- Breakfast: Tropical Breakfast Pie – 5
- Lunch: Beef Chili – Slow-Cooker - 4
- Dinner: Oven-Baked Chicken Kebabs – Slow Cooker – 2
- Dinner Side: Creamy Broccoli – Instant Pot - 4

Totals - Day 20: 15

DAY 21:

- Breakfast: Country Cottage Pancakes - 3
- Lunch: Caesar Salad – Instant Pot – 5
- Dinner: Cajun Salmon – 1
- Dinner Side: Rainbow Side Salad - 4

Totals - Day 21: 13

Now, just continue with the same pattern and add up to your daily number of Freestyle points. These are just your basic meals; so, enjoy the rest of the points but use them wisely each day.

Chapter 8: in conclusion

If your lifestyle is so fast-paced that you believe you cannot possibly drag yourself into the kitchen every night of the week and prepare a healthy and nutritious meal; this unique point system is what you have been searching for to assist you in your dieting needs.

It is wise to monitor your points closely while adjusting to the diet plan because there is an 'open window' to overeat. Just remember even though you are eating -0- points, they still contain calories that can add up quickly if you eat too many. Thus, you could put on the pounds and not understand why. It is one of the quirks of the plan, but by following guidelines such as the enclosed 21-day plan; you can enjoy many -0-points.

Now, you have the information, it's time to get busy and prepare a healthy meal without the guilt. Enjoy each deliciously prepared meal!

Index for the recipes

As an additional convenience, as you are preparing your menu; you can use this unique index with the Freestyle points listed for each of the recipe selections.

Chapter 2: Breakfast Favorites

Chapter 3: Lunch Favorites

Poultry

Salads

- Caesar Salad – Instant Pot – 5

- Ham Salad - 2

- Pear & Blue Cheese Salad - 3

- Tuna Salad with Cranberries – Onion & Celery - 3

Soups

- Beef Chili – Slow-Cooker - 4

- Butternut Squash Soup – 1

- Chicken-Parmesan Soup – 3

- Fish & Shrimp Stew - 2

- Lentil Soup – Instant Pot – 1

- Vegetable Soup -0-

Chapter 4 Scrumptious Dinner Choices: Beef – Fish & Seafood

Beef Choices

- Beef & Broccoli Stir-Fry – 3

- Beef & Mushrooms – Slow Cooker – 5

- Jalapeno Popper Burgers – 6

- Spicy Beef & Zucchini Skillet - 6

Fish & Seafood

- Apple Trout – 3
- Cajun Salmon - 1

Chapter 5: scrumptious dinner choices: Pork & poultry

Pork

- Cuban Pork – Instant Pot – 5
- Pork Chops with Creamy Sauce – 5
- Raspberry Pork Chops in the Crock Pot - 8

Poultry

- Cheesy Southwestern Chicken – Slow Cooker -1
- Italian – Balsamic Chicken - 1
- Oven-Baked Chicken Kebabs – Slow Cooker - 2
- Pesto Baked Chicken - 3

Chapter 6: Sides

- Asparagus Sauteed with Bacon – 1
- Brown Sugar Baked Beans – Instant Pot - 2
- Caesar Green Beans – 2
- Creamy Broccoli – Instant Pot - 4
- Fully-Loaded Macaroni & Cheese with Veggies – 6
- Mashed Sweet Potatoes – 2
- Pinto Beans – Crockpot - 0-
- Rainbow Potato Salad – 4
- Roasted Carrots - 2

Chapter 9: Low FODMAP diet FAQ

As we are nearing our time together, hopefully, you are feeling better about starting the low FODMAP diet. While you have learned a lot about the diet, feel free to check back whenever you have a question about the diet. Whether you need a refresher on the benefits of the diet or a reminder of which foods you can and cannot eat, you will be able to find the information here easily.

To finish off, we will hopefully be able to answer any further questions you have about the low FODMAP diet. Simply remember that this diet is going to be specifically tailored up to you. Being diagnosed with IBS or other GI tract issues is not the end of the world. It will take some extra effort, but when your symptoms and discomfort are relieved, you will be thankful you made the choice to start the low FODMAP diet. For now, it is time to answer some more popular questions you may still have.

Q. I am following the low FODMAP diet and still experiencing symptoms, is this the right diet for me?

A. The answer could be yes and no. If you are following the diet and still find yourself with symptoms of IBS, there may be another culprit in your diet. Remember to keep a food diet with you at all times so you can find any triggers you may be missing.

Q. Can I follow the low FODMAP diet as a vegetarian?

A. Absolutely! You can follow this diet whether you are vegan or vegetarian, it will just take a little extra work. You will find in the chapters before there are plenty of choices, so long as the allowed foods are not triggers for your own body. Some good sources of protein for this diet would be chickpeas, tofu, tempeh, and more. If there is a will, there is always a way!

Q. How do I make sure I'm getting enough Fiber?

A. This is one of the bigger concerns for those following the low FODMAP diet, especially if constipation is an issue. Luckily, several good low FODMAP sources can help you keep your fiber intake up. These include chia seeds, brown rice, flax seeds, kiwi, oranges, white potato, rice bran and more. Check out the list provided in the fourth chapter for a longer list.

Q. Should I eat Larger or Smaller Meals on the Low FODMAP Diet?

A. In general, you should try to eat three main meals through your day and to snacks between these meals. If you are still hungry, you can always add in another snack. Remember that portion control is going to be vital while you are on the low FODMAP diet, so this is something you will want to keep in mind when plating your meals.

Q. What is the rule with fats and oils on the Low FODMAP Diet?

A. As a general rule, there are plenty of fats and oils that are low in FODMAPs. However, anything in excess can trigger IBS symptoms. You will want to be especially aware of any condiments or sauces that are oil-based such as salad dressings. Most of the time, these also include high FODMAPs like garlic. Remember to always read the labels before consuming anything. You can also refer to our extended grocery list to see which fats and oils are allowed on the diet.

Q. Can I eat meat on the low FODMAP Diet?

A. Yes and No. Some sources of animal protein such as fish and chicken are low in FODMAPs. However, if the meat is prepared

.

www.ingramcontent.com/pod-product-compliance
Lightning Source LLC
Chambersburg PA
CBHW070935030426
42336CB00014BA/2681